Good

Bones

■

The Complete Guide to Building & Maintaining the Healthiest Bones

Barbara Luke, ScD, MPH, RD

BULL PUBLISHING

Bull Publishing Company
P.O. Box 208
Palo Alto, CA 94302-0208
Phone (650) 322-2855
Fax (650) 327-3300
www.bullpub.com

ISBN 0-923521-44-5

Distributed in the United States by:
Publishers Group West
1700 Fourth Street
Berkeley, CA 94710

Publisher: James Bull
Production: Publication Services
Cover Design: Robb Pawlak, Pawlak Design
Cover Photo: Bruce Plotkin/Tony Stone Images
Back Cover Photo: Lin Goings
Printer: Malloy Lithographing, Inc.

Library of Congress Cataloging-in-Publication Data
Luke, Barbara.
    Good bones : the complete guide to building &
maintaining the healthiest bones / Barbara Luke.
        p. cm.
    Includes bibliographical references and index.
    ISBN 0-923521-44-5
    1. Osteoporosis—Prevention. 2. Bones. 3. Women—
Health and hygiene.   I. Title.
RC931.073L85   1998   98-33849
616.7'16—dc21   CIP

Table of Contents

To my mother, Ruth Eleanor Luke,
my sister, Dianne Pearson,
and my friend, Ronna Cohen Talcott,
for their sweet hearts and good bones!

Acknowledgments

I would like to acknowledge with greatful appreciation the help and encouragement of my dear friends, Ronna Cohen Talcott, Loretta Mackenroth, and Michal Avni for their careful readings of earlier versions of this manuscript and their thoughtful comments.

Introduction

Osteoporosis is of primary concern today in women's health. Over the past ten years national health organizations have raised public awareness of this health problem, offering guidelines and reccomendations for prevention and treatment.

- In 1988, the U.S. Surgeon General wrote, "the prevalence, health consequences, and expense of osteoporosis among Americans make it a compelling public health priority."
- The 1989 revision of the Recommended Dietary Allowances (RDAs) from the Food and Nutrition Board of the National Academy of Sciences included increases in the calcium requirements and changes in the age groupings, both reflecting newer knowledge of the relationship between diet and bone health.
- In 1992, the National Institutes of Health chose osteoporosis, one of the three diseases that pose the greatest threat to the lives and independence of American women, as a major focus of the newly created Women's Health Initiative.
- In 1994, the National Institutes of Health issued higher daily calcium recommendations for all women.
- In 1998, the Food and Nutrition Board issued their most current calcium recommendations, based on the overwhelming evidence linking diet and health.

- The US Department of Health and Human Services' health objectives for the nation for the year 2000 includes improving the calcium content of the average American's diet.

Osteoporosis, an age-related bone disorder characterized by an increased susceptibility to fractures, is the *fourth leading cause of death among American women.* Osteoporosis is a major public health threat for 28 million Americans, 80% of whom are women. According to the National Osteoporosis Foundation, 10 million individuals already have the disease and 18 million more have low bone mass, increasing their risk. Half of all women and one out of eight men over the age of 50 will eventually suffer an osteoporosis-related bone fracture. One out of six women aged 50 and older will fracture her wrist. One-third of women aged 65 and older will experience vertebral fractures, the most common break caused by osteoporosis. More than 1.5 million osteoporotic fractures occur each year in the United States, including more than 300,000 hip fractures. Many women are shocked when they are told by their physicians that they have osteoporosis. Perhaps this is why the National Osteoporosis Foundation refers to this condition as the "silent thief," since it rarely gives any warning signs.

We build bones over a lifetime, and many factors along the way can either help or hinder our *peak bone mass*—the maximum amount of bone we acquire before age-related losses begin. Unlike other books currently on the market, which focus on the woman only during menopause and later, *Good Bones* approaches prevention from the very beginning of life, before birth, and examines risk factors and offers solutions during every stage of the life cycle. Prevention of osteoporosis must begin early—the earlier, the better. Each chapter in *Good Bones* focuses on the proven risk factors for osteoporosis, and the key points are summarized as "Bone Basics." The final chapter, "Putting It All Together: A Game Plan for Women of All Ages," applies the seventeen risk factors in case studies, as *Bone Health Risk Scores.* Although all seventeen risk factors do not carry equal weight, this summary score helps quantify overall risk. A summary score of 3 or less is low risk; a score of 4 is moderate risk; and a score of 5 or greater, is high risk. Keep in mind that the effect of the same risk factor may change substantially at different ages. For example, diet is one of these risk factors, but certainly what a six-year-old girl eats (or doesn't eat!) is different from what her sixteen-year-old sister eats, and very different from the diet of their 36-year-old mother or 56-year-old grandmother. Included in *Good Bones* is practical advice on how to modify your favorite recipes so that they fit today's nutrition guidelines and still keep their taste appeal. Included, too, are nutritionally sound recommendations on how to change your daily diet to ensure a balanced diet that's "bone-healthy" and "heart-healthy."

The loss of bone mass after menopause is an inevitable occurrence, but much can be done both to acquire a greater peak bone mass before and to slow the rate of loss after menopause. Because osteoporosis usually progresses without any signs or symptoms, we may first become aware we have it when a fracture occurs or when we get a routine chest X-ray. More than likely, we may first make the connection when our mothers experience an osteoporotic hip fracture. Although it's never too late to slow its progress, prevention is the best medicine. This translates into ensuring that our children have the healthiest lifestyles possible so that they build strong bones with greater peak bone mass: their best insurance against developing osteoporosis in later years.

Good Bones is an important book for today's woman, with practical information that can be utilized right now, for herself, her family, and for those she loves. Osteoporosis is a major chronic disease in the United States, but it is preventable and treatable if we act now. Prevention is the single most important therapy for this disorder, and *Good Bones* provides the game plan for putting proven prevention into action.

CHAPTER 1

What Are Good Bones and How Do We Get Them?

Bone Basics

- *Bone mass and bone density increase the most during childhood and adolescence.*
- *Half the adult skeleton is formed between the ages of 10 and 20.*
- *The calcium content of bones triples during the adolescent growth spurt.*
- *Bone density continues to increase, although at a slower rate, through our thirties.*
- *The average woman has more than one-third of her life to live after menopause.*
- *Osteoporosis is a leading cause of death among American women.*

Mary, age 48, has just been diagnosed with osteoporosis. She made an appointment to get her bone density measured when her mother, age 73, was hospitalized with an osteoporotic hip fracture. She had heard that a family history of osteoporosis increases a woman's own risk, so she asked her family physician for advice. In addition to measuring her bone density, her physician reviewed her risk factors. This review helped Mary understand why, even before she had gone through menopause, she had developed osteoporosis. Let's look at her history and see whether you can spot the factors which lead to her present poor bone health.

As a preschooler, Mary preferred fruits and vegetables to sweets and pastries. As a young child in grade school, her tastes were still influenced more by her parents than by her peers. She was an active child, ate a well-balanced diet, and grew strong. However, by adolescence she began experimenting with the latest diets, dropping five or six pounds in a week and exercising several hours a day. Mary became fashionably slender, even to the point of being considered skinny. She experienced menarche (the start of monthly menstrual periods) late, at age 16, and her periods were often irregular. She no longer took her mother's advice about diet, subsisting for long periods on diet sodas and pretzels. By the time Mary had finished college and graduate school, she had maintained her slim figure for ten years, although she had improved her diet somewhat, leaning now mostly to vegetarian dishes and occasional dairy products. At age 30, Mary got married and tried to start a family of her own. But because of her low body fat and irregular periods, it was several years before Mary became pregnant, and even with good weight gain, her baby was small and came earlier than expected. Mary could not make enough breast milk for her baby, so for the first year she fed her baby formula. As her daughter grew older, Mary became more aware of nutrition and tried to plan a balanced diet for her family. She still limited her own intake of dairy products, considering them fattening, and she watched her diet carefully, maintaining a weight that was low for her height. Mary's schedule became busier with her daughter now in grade school, and she found little time to exercise. It was when her daughter was in high school that Mary's mother was hospitalized with an osteoporotic hip fracture. Mary thought she might also be at risk too, and, as the results of the bone density tests revealed, at age 48 Mary had osteoporosis.

Does Mary sound familiar? Her situation reflects many of the factors that have set the stage for poor bone health for millions of American women today—bone losses that are difficult to slow and even more difficult to reverse once the damage has been done. We build our bones over a lifetime. Bones are constantly being formed and remodeled, influenced by a combination of genetics, body build, hormonal status, diet, physical activity, and lifestyle factors. During our growing years we increase both the amount of bone in our bodies (*bone mass*) and the amount of calcium and minerals in our bones (*bone density*). After menopause, we all lose bone mass as part of the aging process, but women who have attained a *greater peak bone mass*—a larger amount of bone before these age-related losses begin—are much less likely to develop osteoporosis. Bone mass and bone density increase the most during two critical time periods: *childhood* and *adolescence.* Mary probably had good bone health through childhood, because she was physically active and ate well. She had gotten off to a good start. During adolescence, though, she probably didn't attain as much bone mass as she could have; low body fat, late menarche, and irregular periods all indicate that she had several risk factors for poor bone development at that crucial stage. Her low body fat throughout her reproductive years not only affected her bone health but also resulted in poor growth of her baby before birth and limited Mary's ability to breast-feed. Bone density continues to increase, although at a slower rate, through our twenties and thirties. Mary missed this last chance to improve her bone health by maintaining a very low body weight throughout her adult years, not continuing to exercise, and avoiding calcium-rich dairy products. Even if she reduced or eliminated all her modifiable risk factors now, at age 48, the best she can hope for is to maintain the bone mass she has already achieved. Without taking these actions, she will continue to lose bone mass rapidly as she enters menopause.

Osteoporosis in America

Osteoporosis, an age-related bone disorder characterized by an increased susceptibility to fractures, affects 28 million Americans, 80% of whom are women. Because we are living longer today than at any other time in history, osteoporosis is more common than ever before. The expected life span in the 1990s is 80 years for women and 72 years for men. In other words, women still have more than one-third of their lives to live after menopause. Almost one-half of all women over the age of 50 will experience bone fractures due to osteoporosis. One-third of women aged 65 and older have vertebral (spinal) fractures, the most common break caused by osteoporosis.

Most women don't realize that they might have osteoporosis until a bone fracture occurs, because the disease progresses so slowly. Once a fracture does occur, osteoporosis is a painful, disabling, and often devastating disease. For Mary's mother, her hip fracture meant weeks in the hospital, followed by months of convalescence at home. Even after she returned home, her mobility was limited and her confidence shaken. As we age we lose muscle, and the immobility of major surgery and convalescence can accelerate that loss. Because she is in her seventies, Mary's mother healed much more slowly, and her recovery from surgery took a long time. Even a year later, she felt that she never really regained her strength or her independence.

Bones are formed over a lifetime, with peak bone mass achieved by the late thirties or early forties. Age-related bone loss is a universal phenomenon, beginning around menopause. Peak bone mass, therefore, is a crucial factor in a woman's ultimate risk of developing osteoporosis. Because of these factors, the emphasis of this book is on women and how we can improve our bone health and reduce our risks for osteoporosis at every stage in the life cycle.

What Are the Risk Factors for Osteoporosis?

You probably know that children under age 12 need calcium every day for their growing bones. But did you know that between the ages of 10 and 20 half of their adult skeleton is formed, or that during the adolescent growth spurt the amount of calcium in their bones triples? Or that your own bones may still be growing throughout your thirties?

Bones are remodeled throughout our lifetimes, with continual loss and addition. Factors that accelerate the rate of loss or slow the rate of addition increase our risk of osteoporosis, such as extreme weight loss, complete bed rest, calcium-poor diets, physical inactivity, smoking, and alcohol use. Reducing these *modifiable risks* at each stage of life is the best investment in strong, healthy bones—*good bones*—at every age. Hormonal status is another critical risk factor for bone health, and is as important for women experiencing menopause as it is for their adolescent daughters. Very low body fat, resulting from high levels of physical activity or from starvation diets, can delay menarche (the initiation of regular menstrual periods), giving your 16-year-old daughter the bone health of her 70-year-old grandmother. Both are lacking sufficient hormones to maintain good bone health.

Diet and physical activity are central to bone health at every stage of the life cycle, but certainly both of these factors change as we age. Most of us don't eat the same foods and in the same amounts as we did when we were children, nor are we as active as we were then. Other things also change as we age, including the development of chronic diseases such as high blood pressure. Medications taken for such diseases can alter bone health and therefore are important to consider when evaluating your overall risk. For a woman, the reproductive years, including the number of pregnancies, whether she breast-fed her baby and for how long, and her prenatal diet, can play an important role in her subsequent bone health as she enters menopause. For an older woman, whether she took oral contraceptives before menopause and for how long, as well as her lifelong dietary habits, can all affect her current bone health.

Some risk factors, such as your racial or ethnic background, are *nonmodifiable*—they can't be changed. The greater your nonmodifiable risks, the more important it is to make every effort to reduce as many of your *modifiable risks* as possible. Although every woman's overall risk for osteoporosis increases with age, it is never too late to improve your bone health and decrease your risks for developing osteoporosis. The practical information and recommendations in *Good Bones* will help you achieve this goal.

This book is organized around the fifteen major risk factors for bone health and discusses each in the context of the life cycle: the prenatal and infancy stages, childhood, adolescence, young adulthood, middle age, and older adulthood. Case studies illustrate how the risk factors influence bone health. Each chapter explains how to evaluate your level of risk for each factor and how to reduce or eliminate those factors that are modifiable.

The goal of *Good Bones* is prevention. In addition to the recommendations for reducing your risks, this book will discuss the issues of hormone replacement therapy—probably the single most important, yet controversial, method of preventing osteoporosis in postmenopausal women. We will look at a variety of ways to improve the calcium content of your diet, including a dozen ways to boost your calcium intake today. Calcium supplements are an increasingly important alternative to dietary calcium for safeguarding our bone health. Chapter 7, "The Prescription Factors," explains how to choose the right calcium supplements for you, and when and how to take them to maximize their effect.

Why This Book Is Important Now

Osteoporosis, along with heart disease and cancer, is one of the leading threats to the lives and independence of American women. It is a leading cause of death among women in the United States today. In 1988, the Surgeon General of the United States declared the prevention of osteoporosis a "compelling public health priority." The prevention of osteoporosis is a major part of the National Institute of Health's 1992 Women's Health Initiative. Increasing the calcium content in the average American's diet is one of the health objectives for the nation for the year 2000 of the U.S. Department of Health and Human Services. The latest revision of the National Academy of Sciences' Recommended Dietary Allowances (RDAs) included increases in the calcium requirements and changes in the age groupings, both reflecting newer knowledge of the relationship between dietary calcium and bone health. In 1997, the latest calcium recommendations from the Institute of Medicine reflect the importance of this nutrient in bone health. Osteoporosis is one of the chronic diseases, like heart disease and cancer, that become evident in adulthood but have their origins in childhood and adolescence. Many factors contribute to the development and severity of osteoporosis, but if they are reduced or eliminated while bones are still forming and even afterwards, the risk of osteoporosis can be greatly reduced. Ideally, prevention should begin during childhood, with a good diet and healthy habits. At each stage of the life cycle there are many opportunities to improve peak bone mass and reduce the risk of osteoporosis. This book is for you, your family, friends, older relatives, and younger relatives. The practical advice in *Good Bones* will help you improve your own bone health and the health of those you love—regardless of their ages.

How Do Bones Develop and What Affects Them?

Before you can take charge of your bone health, you need to know some basic information about your bones and how they work. This next section gives you those basics, as well as an introduction to the seventeen most important risk factors that influence your bone health at every stage of the life cycle.

How Your Living Skeleton Works

Bones are living, renewing, vital components of the human body that reflect a combination of lifelong dietary and exercise habits, as well as our individual, unique genetic heritage. Bones serve two major functions: one *structural* and one *biochemical.* The structural function is the one that's most familiar: to provide the structural framework of our bodies; to allow us to move, walk, and run; and to protect our vital internal organs and tissues. The second function, which is equally as important but not as obvious, is as a reservoir of calcium and other minerals, storing and releasing them as part of the delicate balance of metabolism that's maintained 24 hours every day. The bones in our bodies are wonderfully suited for the jobs they do. Our long bones, which do most of the weight bearing, are built with a dense outer layer, called *cortical* or *compact* bone, and a spongy inner layer, called *trabecular* or *porous* bone. The bones in our bodies that act as shock absorbers or that must be flexible, such as the ribs, are made up mostly of spongy trabecular bone. Made up of about 70% minerals, bones are primarily calcium, phosphorus, and magnesium, and about 30% water and connective tissue protein (collagen). Similar to the structural protein in tendons and skin, collagen is as strong as steel ounce for ounce.

The skeleton smoothly orchestrates its structural and biochemical functions during the life cycle, keeping us sitting, standing, walking, and running, while efficiently maintaining the proper balance of minerals in our bloodstream within a very narrow normal range. You may think of calcium as just a "structural" mineral—

only needed to build bones—but it has many other vital functions, not least of which is to keep your heart beating! A constant, steady supply of calcium in the bloodstream is necessary for muscles to contract (to get your skeleton moving), for cells to reproduce and heal, for enzymes to function, and for metabolism to proceed—in other words, for life itself. So calcium is at the very heart of both our physical and biochemical lives.

It's Always Time To Remodel

Bones are constantly being formed and resorbed during our lifetimes by the actions of two specialized types of bone cells. *Osteoblasts* create the bone framework of collagen, and they attract calcium and other minerals to mineralize or strengthen bones by increasing its density. **Osteoclasts** are the bone cells responsible for bone breakdown, or resorption; they dissolve bone and release calcium and minerals into the bloodstream. The key players influencing bone formation and resorption are hormones, primarily **parathormone** (from the parathyroid gland), **calcitonin** (from the thyroid gland), **calcitriol** (the active form of vitamin D), and **estrogen** (from the ovaries); other sex hormones and growth factors also influence bone health at various stages during the life cycle.

The rates of bone formation and bone resorption vary depending on our age. For example, the turnover rate for bone calcium is 100% per year during infancy and slows to about 10% per year for adults. The renewal rates for compact bone and trabecular bone are influenced by the amount of stress and strain imposed on the skeleton and by the levels of hormones and growth factors. This means that during early childhood the skeleton is completely rebuilt in a year, whereas over that same time period only about one-tenth of an adult's skeleton is new bone. Building bone is especially important during the critical periods of childhood and adolescence, because this rate of renewal and growth slows as we age.

Balance Is Everything

Bone mineral content increases during growth, when the mass of the skeleton is increasing. *Bone mineral density* increases as bone is being mineralized (when calcium and other minerals are being deposited into the collagen framework), which occurs most rapidly during the first three years of life and during adolescence. When more calcium is being absorbed during digestion than is being lost in the urine or via the gastrointestinal tract, calcium is being added to the skeleton, indicating *positive calcium balance.* When more calcium is being excreted or mobilized than is being absorbed, calcium is being taken from the skeleton, indicating *negative calcium balance.* At all ages, from infancy through young adulthood, calcium balance comes closer to zero and becomes constant at higher dietary levels, while at lower levels calcium balance is highly correlated with dietary intake. This threshold of necessary dietary calcium, which parallels increasing age, is the amount of calcium needed to ensure the best skeletal retention of calcium. Research indicates that for nearly every age through young adulthood, this threshold level of dietary calcium is higher than current dietary recommendations and substantially higher than current dietary levels of intake.

When we are habitually in negative calcium balance over many years, bones become thin and fragile. The structure of bone becomes so weak and damaged that it cannot support normal weight bearing. Eventually, with continued loss of bone density, we enter the *critical fracture zone,* when bones can fracture or become deformed in response to ordinary stresses in daily life. This means that you can fracture a bone by just tripping on an uneven pavement, lifting a bag of groceries, bumping into a kitchen counter, raking leaves, or even sneezing. These fractures can occur without attracting much notice, or they can occur dramatically. Because of its more rapid rate of turnover, trabecular bone is much more susceptible to loss and the development of osteoporosis. *One of the most common sites of bone loss is the spinal column,* the *backbone,* which is predominantly made of the spongy trabecular bone. Spontaneous crush fractures of the vertebrae can lead to curvature of the spine (known as dowager's hump), loss of height, and chronic pain. These types of osteoporotic fractures can occur without symptoms or with sudden, intense back pain. Fractures of the hip (especially at the neck of the femur, or thigh bone) and the radius (the forearm bone on the thumb side) are a common consequence of osteoporosis, since these areas have a high content of trabecular bone. For this reason, bone density—the amount of calcium per unit of bone—is most frequently measured in the distal (wrist end) third of the radius shaft; at the level of the second through fourth vertebrae of the lumbar spine (L2-L4), and in the proximal (hip end) femur (see Figure 1). Because many women

FIGURE 1
Common sites of osteoporotic fractures
■ ■

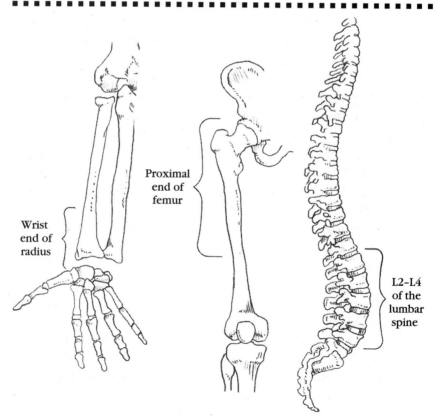

Wrist
end of
radius

Proximal
end of
femur

L2-L4
of the
lumbar
spine

spend about half their lives dangerously close to or within the critical fracture zone, whereas men rarely enter it before age 80, osteoporosis is predominantly a woman's disease.

Measuring Bone Health: The Inside Story

Until recently, measuring bone density (the amount of calcium per unit of bone) has not been considered a routine procedure. Few hospitals or clinics have the appropriate equipment, and even when they do, this test may not be covered by health insurance. But without such measures we don't know how healthy (or unhealthy) our bones really are. Bone mineral density tests measure bone density in the spine, wrist, hip, heel, or hand. These tests are safe, painless, and noninvasive and can detect low bone density before a fracture occurs, confirm the diagnosis of osteoporosis, and help monitor bone changes when performed yearly. To locate a bone mineral testing center near you, call 1-800-464-6700.

Hormones, nutrients, and other by-products of bone metabolism can be measured in the blood and urine to help complete the overall picture of your bone health. These substances are referred to as biochemical markers, and they help your physician determine whether there are any other reasons besides osteoporosis contributing to bone loss. Biochemical markers can also indicate the rate of bone turnover; depending on your age, these results are interpreted differently. For example, high levels of these biochemical markers during adolescence reflect the accelerated skeletal growth that normally occurs around puberty. After menopause, high levels of these markers indicate accelerated bone loss.

As women become more aware of the need to have their bone density measured, particularly as they enter menopause, and more physicians begin to monitor the bone health of women, these tests will probably become more accessible and affordable. Until that time, though, your next best option is to assess your own risk factors, discuss them with your doctor, and modify those you can to build good bones at every age.

The Seventeen Risk Factors for Every Age

There are seventeen major factors that increase your risk for osteoporosis. Their relative importance depends on your age—the single most important factor. Bone loss is a normal part of the aging process, but we can slow that loss by reducing or eliminating risk factors throughout each stage of the life cycle. The risk factors I'm going to discuss are not clear-cut but are related and often overlap. For example, if you are small-boned, you have a higher risk for developing osteoporosis, but your body build was basically genetically determined. Family history is another risk factor, and you probably have a body build that is similar to your mother's or grandmother's. Physical activity, level of body fat, and hormonal status are also linked. With high levels of physical activity we can lose substantial amounts of body fat, which in turn can result in hormonal imbalances, menstrual irregularities, and an increased risk for osteoporosis. Let's look at the seventeen most important categories of risk for developing osteoporosis and what we can do to reduce or eliminate those that are modifiable. These categories are shown in Table 1.

TABLE 1

■■■■■■■■■■■■■■■■■■■■■■■■■■■■■■■

	Risk Categories	Risk Factors
Hereditary Factors	Race	Asian or Caucasian
	Family history	+Family history
Women-Only Factors	Age at menarche	Menarche at age 14 or older
	Menstrual cycles	Irregular
	Age at menopause	Menopause at age 45 or younger
	Total reproductive years	30 years or less
Body Shape Factors	Body build	Small-boned
	Proportion of fat to muscle	High fat/low muscle
	Weight	Underweight (BMI < 19.8)
Physical Factors	Exercise	Inactive
Prescription Factors	Hormonal status	Estrogen-deficient
	Certain medications	
Lifestyle Factors	Smoking	Smoker
	Alcohol	>one drink/day for women
		>two drinks/day for men
Nutrient Factors	Protein	High protein
	Sodium	High sodium
	Calcium	Low calcium
Bone Health Risk Score		*

*Three or fewer risk factors = low risk.
 Four risk factors = moderate risk.
 Five or more risk factors = high risk.

CHAPTER 2

The Age Factor

The Most Important Factor

Bone Basics:

- *The bones of adults are five times more densely mineralized with calcium than are those of infants.*
- *Bone density increases the most during the first three years of life and late puberty.*
- *More than one-third of the adult bone mass is acquired during adolescence.*
- *Within five to seven years after menopause, women can lose as much as 20 percent of femoral bone.*
- *Without hormone replacement therapy, by age 60 most women have lost 25 percent of their bone mass; by age 70, this figure has risen to 50 percent.*

Age is the single most important factor in your risk for developing osteoporosis. The relative contributions of all your risk factors are influenced by your age when they occur. For example, a deficiency of estrogen during adolescence (as caused by low body fat and high physical activity) can have a devastating effect on the growing skeleton. At age 50, the deficiency of estrogen accompanying menopause still adversely affects the skeleton, but to a lesser extent. By age 75, the relative contribution of estrogen deficiency to the risk of osteoporosis is much less compared to other risk factors. Our bone density (and therefore our risk for osteoporosis) is a cumulative index of our unique risk factors, both past and present. Risk factors that occur during childhood and adolescence may contribute as much to lifetime fracture risk as aging and menopause.

What happens as we age that increases our risk? First, our bodies become less efficient in absorbing calcium from our diets. Absorption of this essential mineral is highest during the first three years of life and during adolescence, when bones are growing most rapidly in both size and density. For individuals younger than about age 20, the body can adapt to a lower calcium intake by increasing the efficiency of calcium absorption. This process is controlled by the hormone calcitriol (the active form of vitamin D). With increasing age, this process becomes less efficient. Age-related decreases in calcium absorption can begin as early as age 30 or as late as age 60. The body's decreased absorption of calcium may result directly from changes in the process of absorption, or indirectly, as a result of decreased production of calcitriol by the kidneys. Second, the hormonal changes that accompany aging, primarily the deficiency in estrogen that occurs with menopause, cause calcium to be released from bone into the bloodstream. As a result, parathyroid hormone and calcitriol levels fall, which in turn reduces calcium absorption in the intestine. Third, the ability of bone cells to regenerate new bone as we age also changes. Even when our diets contain adequate amounts of calcium, the number and efficiency of osteoblasts (the bone-generating cells) decrease with age.

Does this mean we should just throw up our hands and give in to the inevitable? Of course not, but it does mean you should be aware that age itself is your most important nonmodifiable risk. The older you get, the more important it becomes to try to reduce or eliminate as many of your modifiable factors as you can.

Prenatal and Infancy Periods

Before birth and through the first year of life, bones are being built at a steady rate. Before birth, the bones of the developing baby are already being formed by eight weeks after conception, with upper and lower limbs (including toes and fingers) well formed at this point. Although the amount of calcium in the fetal bones is small during early pregnancy, this period is critical for bone development. The use of certain medications and drinking alcohol during this period can result in permanent birth defects. By the middle of pregnancy (about 20 weeks), minerals have begun to be deposited in the fetal bone matrix, with the highest rate of mineralization occuring during the last eight weeks before birth.

Calcium, phosphorus, and magnesium are the main minerals in bone development. Calcium is the most abundant mineral, with 98% of the body's stores present in the bones at any age. Compared to those of infants, the bones of adults are about five times more densely mineralized with calcium. More than 80% of the body's phosphorus is contained in the bones, and as with calcium, the total amount increases with age. Adults have about four times the body content of phosphorus compared to infants. On a weight basis, calcium and phosphorus are present in bone in a ratio of about 2:1. More than 60% of the body's magnesium is stored in our bones; as with calcium and phosphorus, the body content of this mineral increases with age, nearly doubling from infancy to adulthood. At birth, boy and girl infants have comparable bone mineral densities; not until later in childhood do they begin to differ.

At birth one of the biggest risk factors that can interfere with normal bone development is *being born prematurely*—three or more weeks early. In the United States, prematurity affects more than 400,000 newborns every year. Most of the unborn baby's calcium (about 30 grams) is deposited in the bones during the last two months before birth; therefore, if born early, these infants have lower bone mineral content than their full-term nurserymates. These babies need special formulas and feedings to help their new bones catch up. For children born very premature (more than six weeks early), it may take as long as three years for their bones to catch up to their full-term nurserymates. In addition, if a newborn, particularly if born premature, has any digestive problems that interfere with calcium absorption, bone growth slows down. Once the digestive problems have been remedied, bone growth quickly recovers, usually making up for lost time. The lower bone mineral content of premature infants does not persist into childhood; bone mineral content is most strongly related to the child's current body weight.[1]

Premature infants fed breast milk have an adequate growth rate but decreased bone mineral content. Breast milk lacks sufficient levels of calcium and phosphorus to support bone growth and mineralization for premature infants; for this reason it needs to be fortified to meet the special needs of these infants. Enriched infant formulas have also been shown to support good bone growth among premature babies, resulting in bone mineral density comparable to those of babies born at term as early as nine months and no later than two years of age.[2-6] Infants that are born small for their gestational age (less than the 10th percentile), even if they are born at term, have a lower bone mineral content compared to appropriately grown infants (see Figure 1).[7-9] Because calcium is ac-

FIGURE 1

Percentages of birthweight for gestational age (SGA, AGA, and LGA)

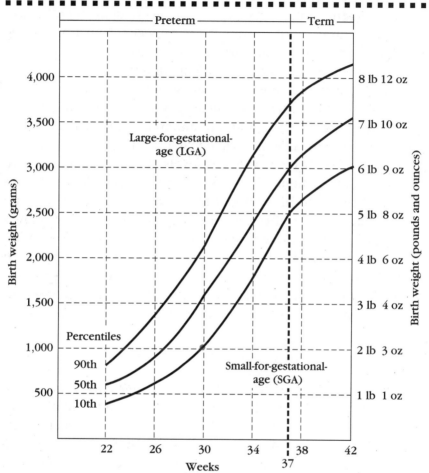

tively transported from the mother to the baby by the placenta, researchers believe the same factors which cause a baby to be born small are also responsible for the decreased supply of calcium.[10] As with premature infants, with fortified formulas or enriched breast milk the bones of these infants can easily catch up in no time at all.

Infancy is one of the most critical nutritional periods of the life cycle. Growth during the first year of life is more rapid than at any other period after birth. Because of this rapid growth, a constant and adequate supply of essential nutrients is vital. In the absence of adequate essential nutrients, clinical signs of nutritional deficiencies appear sooner in infants than in any other age group and have more serious consequences. Nutrition during this stage can affect health throughout life. At birth, the "reliable" steady source of nutrients, including minerals and vitamin D, ceases. The newborn must now obtain nutrients from his or her own diet. All of the calcium-regulating hormones are functioning at the time of birth. The amount of minerals available depends on the feedings, with breast milk considered the optimal choice. Breast milk contains relatively low levels of minerals compared to cow's milk, but its composition is ideally suited for the newborn's needs. Calcium and phosphorus are present in a ratio of 2:1, and more than 80% of the calcium present is absorbed. Cow's milk–based and soy-based infant formulas, which have a higher mineral content and a calcium-to-phosphorus ratio of 1.5:1, both provide adequate amounts of both calcium and phosphorus. Most healthy infants born at term can adjust to a wide range of calcium-to-phosphorus ratios in their diets.

Vitamin D: The Sunshine Factor

An important factor in infant nutrition is the *vitamin D status* of the infant at birth, which in turn is dependent on the mother's vitamin D status. The active form of vitamin D regulates calcium and phosphorus metabolism in three ways: (1) by increasing absorption from the gastrointestinal tract; (2) by regulating reabsorption by the kidneys; and (3) by mobilizing bone sources. All forms of vitamin D, whether transferred from mother to her unborn baby, from diet, or as produced in the skin on exposure to sunlight, have the same effect in the body. The mother's vitamin D levels are dependent on the season of the birth, her sun exposure, and her dietary intake of vitamin D. Infants born in summer have been found to have significantly lower bone mineral content than those born in winter; researchers suggest that the lower bone mineral content among summer-born infants is related to reduced maternal vitamin D status in the preceding winter months.[11]

The half-life of vitamin D is three weeks, which means that infants born with sufficient levels can go for several weeks before requiring either sun exposure, to produce vitamin D in the skin, or supplements. Significant differences in vitamin D status have been shown among breast-fed infants with and without vitamin D supplementation, and in infants fed milk-based and soy-based formulas. For many years infant formula, as well as cow's milk, has been fortified with vitamin D (400 International Units, IU, per quart). Levels of vitamin D are low in breast milk, although they can be increased with a supplement. Breast-fed infants receiving 400 IU of vitamin D as a supplement have blood levels comparable to those of infants receiving 400 IU in their formulas. Even infants who were born with very low blood levels of vitamin D soon achieve normal levels when supplemented.

With adequate vitamin D (from supplements or exposure to sunshine), breast milk supports bone mineralization, at least for the first six months of life. After six months, the phosphorus content of breast milk could limit bone mineralization in infants fed exclusively by this method. Introduction of phosphorus-rich foods (such as cereals) in exclusively breast-fed infants after the age of 6 months is important for mineral balance and good bone development. Infant formulas provide adequate nutrition for bone mineralization throughout the first year of life.

Childhood

Today's children are taller and heavier than those of even a generation ago. Although stature is genetically determined, environmental factors, such as illnesses and the daily diet, influence genetic expression. The eradication of many diseases, including those of nutritional origin, and improvements in the quality and quantity of the average diet have permitted growth during childhood to reach maximal levels of the genetic potential of the individual. During the ages of 2–10, growth continues at a gradual, steady rate, and dramatic changes begin to occur. Much of the characteristic fat present during infancy and early childhood is lost, muscles become stronger, and bones lengthen and increase in density. New bone is first modeled in cartilage and then transformed into bone by mineralization. This growth occurs in specialized areas of cartilage at the ends of the long bones, called the ***epiphyseal plates*** (see Figure 2). As new bone is laid down at the plates, bones lengthen. The width of the epiphyseal plates is proportional to the rate of growth. Linear bone growth continues as long as the epiphyses are separated from the shaft of the bone. When the epiphyses unite with the shaft of the bone (closure of the epiphyseal plates), linear bone growth ceases. The epiphyseal plates of the bones close in a set sequence, with the last epiphyses closing just after puberty. The typical age at which each of the epiphyses closes is known, and because of this, the bone age of an individual can be found by using X-rays to determine which epiphyses are open and which have already closed.

FIGURE 2
Epiphyseal plates

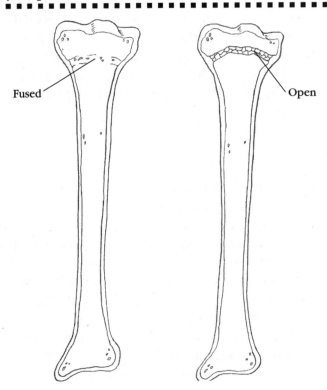

Fused

Open

In the absence of major illnesses, and with adequate exercise and a balanced diet, most children develop strong bones as they grow through childhood, with the strongest correlations to age, height, and body weight. Bone mineral densities increase annually during childhood, but the highest rates of increase are during the first three years of life and during late puberty.[12] Before the age of 4, bone mineral content does not differ among children by race or gender; after this age, though, boys have higher values than girls, and black children have higher values than white or Asian children.

Adolescence

During adolescence (age 10–18 years) the story gets more complicated. Ideally, girls should grow about 10 inches during these years, with bone density increasing by 50–60% and total bone mineral content increasing by 133%. More than one-third of the adult skeletal mass is acquired during adolescence. By age 20, girls have attained nearly 90% of the bone mass of their premenopausal mothers. This rapid growth in both bone mass and bone density is triggered by a flood of hormones and growth factors: the adolescent growth spurt. Almost overnight, these amazing transformations turn girls to young women, preparing their bodies for adulthood. One of the hallmarks that these wonderfully orchestrated processes are taking place is the start of the monthly menstrual periods, *menarche.* Monthly periods indicate that the normal cyclic hormonal changes are occurring, and the levels of these hormones, particularly estrogen, are sufficient to protect the calcium that has been and will be stored in the bones. When menarche is delayed, because of vigorous physical activity, very low body weight, or both—there is no rise in estrogen levels, and calcium that has already been deposited can be lost from the bones.

Adulthood

From adolescence through the mid-thirties, bones continue to grow, but at a slower pace. With regular exercise, a balanced diet, regular monthly periods, and maintenance of normal body weight and adequate percentage of body fat, calcium balance favors deposition, and we continue to acquire bone mass. Although it varies from woman to woman, generally by the time we reach our fortieth birthday we have achieved our lifetime *peak bone mass,* the maximum amount of bone present before age-related losses begin. After about age 40, women begin to slowly lose bone mass, at the rate of less than 1% per year. Although bone is still being remodeled, the balance shifts, and more bone is broken down than is being built up. This slow loss of bone mass continues until we go through menopause, when the rate of loss increases dramatically.

> *Emily is 54 years of age. Last year she began to get hot flashes and night sweats—symptoms that she was going through menopause. Her periods began to be irregular and were shorter and lighter when they did occur. Emily has been physically active all her life, from tennis in high school to jogging during her thirties and forties. Recently she has added cycling to her list, and tries to include some physical activity at least three times a week. She is 5'4" tall, weighs 138 pounds, and has 26% body fat. Ever since childhood she has been a milk drinker, although she has switched from lowfat to skim as she got older. To this day she drinks several quarts a week.*

> *Emily's sister, Lorraine, is 69 years of age. Lorraine went through menopause 15 years ago, at about the same age as Emily is now. They may be sisters, but they are as different as day and night. Lorraine never participated in sports, and always avoided milk. She is also 5'4" tall, but weighs 118 pounds and has 18% body fat. Although both sisters began hormone replacement therapy around menopause, Lorraine has already had several osteoporotic fractures, including a fractured hip last year when she was bumped by a shopping cart in the grocery store.*

As sisters, Emily and Lorraine share the same genetic risk factors for osteoporosis. But because of lifetime differences in both physical activity and diet, their risks for osteoporosis now are very different. Emily is at much lower risk, especially if she continues her program of physical activity and her several-quart-a-week milk habit. These sisters probably began menopause with very different peak bone masses, and as age-related losses occurred, Lorraine soon entered the critical fracture zone and suffered the consequences.

As we enter menopause, our risk for developing osteoporosis increases greatly. With the sudden drop in the bone-protecting hormone estrogen as well as in other hormones, we can lose as much as 2–8% of vertebral bone and as much as 20% of femoral bone within the first 5–7 years after menopause, according to figures from the National Osteoporosis Foundation. This rapid loss occurs through increased calcium losses in the urine and increased bone breakdown, in response to the sudden decline in estrogen. In addition, the ability of the body to absorb calcium decreases. These three sources of decreased calcium—increased urinary losses, increased bone breakdown, and decreased calcium absorption—cannot be reversed by diet alone; the hormonal imbalance must be corrected, too (see Chapter 7, "The Prescription Factors"). By age 60 many women have lost more than 25% of their bone mass and have set the stage for osteoporotic fractures. Although the rate of bone loss slows after that age, by the time many women reach age 70 they may have lost as much as half of their lifetime peak bone mass. This means that many women in their seventies are within the critical fracture zone and are vulnerable to sustaining fractures from the ordinary stresses in daily life. Although the risk for all osteoporotic fractures increases with age, the incidence of wrist fractures generally increases during the fifties, vertebral fractures during the sixties, and hip fractures during the seventies.

Even though the rate of bone loss slows after age 60, the bone that is remodeled is structurally less dense and sturdy. Calcium absorption by the body continues to decline, and the levels of all hormones continue to fall with age. Muscle mass and strength also decrease, making us even more susceptible to accidental falls and fractures. Our bones can become so fragile that ordinary activities of daily living can increase our risk of sustaining a fracture, and exercises that were therapeutic years before have now become too dangerous. Perhaps the worst consequence of osteoporosis is the disability it imposes, with the loss of independence and impaired quality of life.[13] This is particularly true for vertebral fractures, which occur earlier and affect more women than do hip fractures.

The rate of bone loss among women in their sixties and seventies averages 0.5–1.0% per year and may be as high as 3% per year by the time they reach their eighties. Age-related bone loss can be greatly reduced or even eliminated, and the risk of fractures lowered dramatically, with calcium intakes in the range of 1,500–1,700 mg per day.[14,15] Studies have demonstrated that hip fracture rates are at least 60% lower among elderly women whose lifetime calcium intakes were high.[16,17] The message from all of these studies is that adequate calcium, in combination with other factors, is central to good bone health, and although the sooner the better, it's never too late to take positive actions to improve your bones.

As you can see, age itself is the most important risk factor for osteoporosis. Although we cannot stop the clock, we can reduce or eliminate many of the other risk factors all along the life cycle. The next chapter will discuss the roles of race, ethnicity, and family history—nonmodifiable risks. Although they cannot be changed, these are important factors to consider when viewing your overall risk for osteoporosis. They can also influence the effect of other modifiable risk factors such as diet, physical activity, and lifestyle choices on your bone health at every age.

CHAPTER 3

The Heredity Factors

Race, Ethnicity, and Family History

Bone Basics:

- *By adulthood, black women have 10–15% greater bone density.*

- *Genetic factors explain 90% of the variation in bone mass in the spine and 70% in the hip joint.*

- *There is a strong correlation between the bone masses of mothers and their daughters.*

- *By age 20, a daughter will have attained 90% of her mother's height and bone mass.*

- *A son has a nearly fourfold higher risk of having low bone density if his father has low bone density.*

- *A daughter has more than a fivefold higher risk of having low bone density if her mother has low bone density.*

Even before we are born, we bring a set of factors with us that can either decrease or increase our bone health: our racial and genetic heritage. Although age-related and menopause-related bone losses occur among every racial and ethnic group, all groups are not at equal risk for developing osteoporosis. Light-skinned women are at the highest risk: women whose ancestry originated from northern Europe, the United Kingdom, and the Far East are at much greater risk than those who are of Hispanic, African, or Mediterranean descent. Even at birth, black babies have heavier skeletons than their white nurserymates.[1,2] By adulthood, black women have 10–15% greater bone density, primarily as cortical bone, than do light-skinned women. After menopause, this difference translates into vastly different risks for osteoporotic fractures. For example, by age 65, black women have about 40% as much risk of developing an osteoporotic hip fracture as do their Asian or Caucasian counterparts.[3] By age 80, the lifetime risk of hip fracture for the average black woman is 1 in 20, compared to a 1 in 6 for the average white woman.[4] This difference in bone mineral density is evident even among men, with black men having about 7% greater bone mineral density than white men. Part of this lower risk for osteoporosis stems from racial differences in body content of potassium—a measure of total cellular mass, especially muscle. Generally, black women have a larger muscle mass, perhaps linked to their greater skeletal mass, which in turn partly explains their lower risk for osteoporosis.[5]

The racial influence on bone health is not merely because of differences in skin color. There are also distinct differences in metabolism and physiology, and probably others we have yet to uncover. Bone development is the result of a delicate balance of many factors, including essential nutrients and hormones. Studies around the world have demonstrated distinct metabolic differences between the races, thought to be primarily an evolutionary adaptation to the environment. For example, serum calcitonin, a bone-protecting hormone, is significantly higher in West Indian blacks than in whites.[6] Because of a decreased synthesis of vitamin D in the skin of darker-skinned populations, they have a lower rate of bone turnover and therefore an increased bone mass.[7] These differences, in turn, alter the effects of modifiable factors such as diet and exercise. For example, recent studies show that during adolescence, black girls achieve a higher positive calcium balance than white girls do, because of lower urinary losses of calcium.[8] Adult black women have a slower rate of bone turnover compared to adult white women, reducing their overall risk for osteoporosis after menopause.[9] In addition, black women over the age of 65 have higher levels of *estrone,* the major form of estrogen in postmenopausal women.[10] All of these differences add up to a lower overall risk for osteoporosis for black women compared to their white, Asian, or Hispanic counterparts.

Asian women are at highest risk for osteoporosis, in part because of their smaller bone mass compared to other racial groups. Improving modifiable risk factors, such as diet and physical activity, can greatly reduce this racial risk. For example, Eskimos have a lower bone mineral content than whites, and they begin losing it at an earlier age and at a faster rate.[11,12] This effect is believed to be related more to a diet high in phosphorus and protein than to a genetic predisposition (see Chapter 9, "The Nutrient Factors"). A nearly universal finding, in studies of populations around the world, is that higher dietary calcium intake is associated with better bone health, particularly among women.[13]

Like Mother, Like Daughter

We often forget the fact that we inherit much of our body build, body weight, and proportions of body fat. Whether we like it or not, we most likely resemble our parents in our physical appearance. Studies have confirmed this observation, showing significant correlations between mothers, daughters, and grandmothers in height and triceps skinfold thicknesses (a measure of body fat).[14] Another nonbiological factor related to heritage and family is our diets: what we eat, at least during our childhood years, is influenced by our parents, who in turn were influenced by their parents.

You may have your father's quick wit and your mother's winning smile, but your parents have also given you something else—the hereditary foundation of your bone health. Genetic factors contribute substantially to peak bone mass, as demonstrated in studies of twins, of mothers and daughters, and of parents and children. These studies generally conclude that hereditary factors exert a greater influence earlier in life, during periods of growth such as childhood and early adulthood, whereas environmental factors (including diet, physical activity, and hormonal status) exert their influence over the entire life span, and particularly after menopause among women. Studies of identical twins suggest that the proportion of the variation in bone mass that can be explained by genetic factors is approximately 90% in the lumbar spine and 70% in the femoral neck (hip joint). [15-17] In studies of mothers and daughters, who share half their genes, this correlation is about 45% and 35%, respectively. Most studies have reported a positive correlation between the bone mass of mothers and daughters, but some of this familial resemblance may be due to common lifestyle habits that are related to bone health, such as lifelong exercise habits or milk consumption.[14,18-20] Studies of mother-daughter pairs among postmenopausal mothers with osteoporosis and their premenopausal daughters have provided even more insight into this relationship. One study reported that daughters of women with osteoporosis have reduced bone mass in the lumbar spine and femoral neck.[21] Others have suggested that the nature of inheritance of bone mass may have at least two components: one influencing the level of peak bone mass, and another related to the rate of bone loss at menopause.[22]

Peak bone mass, bone size, and bone density in young women are strongly influenced by genetic contributions not only from their mothers, but from their fathers as well. In studies of parents and their children, we have learned even more about the effect of nature (genetics) versus nurture (environment) on bone health. One large study of 129 families found bone mineral density to be positively correlated with body weight and height in all family members and with physical activity in fathers and sons.[23] These researchers concluded that a son had a 3.8-fold higher risk of having a low bone mineral density if his father had a low bone mineral density, and a daughter had a 5.1-fold higher risk if her mother had a low bone mineral density.

Genetic factors are very important in your overall risk for osteoporosis. Look to your mother and grandmother to get some idea of your own genetic future. If they did not reduce their own modifiable risks, though, particularly the hormonal changes after menopause, those genetic effects will be magnified. By age 20, your daughter will have attained 90% of your height and bone mass. Genetics may influence not only how fast we lose bone after menopause but how much bone mass we attain before those inevitable age-related losses even begin: our peak bone mass. Postmenopausal osteoporosis may result partly from a relatively low peak bone mass as well as excessive bone loss after menopause. Genetic factors may also influence the susceptibility of our bones to environmental factors, such as diet, smoking, and alcohol. Maybe we should change that old adage, "You can choose your friends, but not your relatives," to "You can choose your diet, but not your genes."

Current scientific evidence supports a strong hereditary contribution to the development of peak bone mass.[24,25] Environmental factors, such as diet (including calories, protein, calcium, and vitamin D), physical activity, and hormonal factors each exert separate effects, though to a lesser extent than the genetic contribution to bone mass. Although race and genetics are nonmodifiable factors, they are important to consider when assessing your overall risk. In the next chapter we will see how the women-only factors, from menarche to menopause, fit into the overall picture of bone health.

CHAPTER 4

The Women-Only Factors

From Menarche to Menopause

Bone Basics:

- *Women lose 25% of their bone mass (750 grams of their 3,000-gram skeleton).*

- *Men lose 12% of their bone mass (450 grams of their 4,000-gram skeleton).*

- *Women lose about 35% of cortical bone and 50% of trabecular bone.*

- *Women who had delayed menarche have a threefold increased risk for fractures during and after menopause.*

- *Irregular menstrual cycles increase the risk for stress fractures, scoliosis, and vertebral fractures before menopause.*

- *Oral contraceptive use can increase bone mass by as much as 2–3%.*

- *Breast-feeding doubles a woman's daily calcium losses.*

Women are at much greater risk of developing osteoporosis than men for several reasons. First, we have about 25% less peak bone mass compared to men. Second, we lose bone at a faster rate and more dramatically in our fifties (around menopause) than our male counterparts, due to the abrupt decline in the bone-saving hormones. For example, after about age 50, we lose 25% of our bone mass, or about 750 grams of our 3,000-gram skeleton, whereas men lose about 12% of their bone mass, or about 450 grams of their 4,000-gram skeleton. During our lifetimes, we will lose about 35% of our cortical bone and about 50% of our trabecular bone. During the first five to seven years after menopause, 2–8% of vertebral bone is lost and 20% of femoral bone is lost. Third, the period of accelerated bone loss for men occurs about a decade later than it does for women. Therefore, peak bone mass, the maximum amount of bone present before age-related loss begins, is of vital importance, particularly for women. Nonetheless, men account for 20% of all individuals who develop osteoporosis.

When men under the age of 75 develop this condition, it is most likely due to an underlying problem such as excessive alcohol consumption, gastrointestinal surgery, low levels of testosterone, or medications for asthma or inflammatory disease. As with women, osteoporosis among men is often not detected until a fracture occurs or low bone density is revealed on a routine X-ray.

Because of the much greater incidence of osteoporosis among women, this chapter will focus on our specific health issues, including the menstrual cycle, oral contraceptives, treatments for endometriosis, pregnancy and breast-feeding, hysterectomy, menopause, and, after menopause, the cumulative effect of the reproductive years.

Menarche and Menstrual Cycles

Menarche, the start of regular monthly menstrual cycles, is the primary woman's health issue during adolescence. The right combination of body weight and adequate body fat triggers hormonal changes, which in turn initiates regular menstrual periods.[1] It has been suggested that girls need to attain 17% body fat for menarche to occur and 22% body fat to maintain regular menstrual cycles.[2] Below a threshold level of body fat or body weight, menarche and menstrual cycles are adversely affected, but this exact threshold may vary from individual to individual and may be additionally influenced by other factors, such as physical activity and stress levels. A *delay in menarche* (when regular menstrual periods begin at age 14 or later), due to vigorous physical activity, low body fat, or other disturbances of hormonal balance, is a risk factor for current and long-term poor bone health. Adolescence is one of the two most important periods in the life cycle for rapid bone growth, with as much as 37% of the adult bone mass acquired during this period. Immediate and long-term adverse consequences can result when less bone mass is acquired during this critical period. Studies have shown significantly higher rates of stress fractures during the reproductive years, and lower bone mass, bone density, and a greater than threefold increased risk of bone fractures during and after menopause among women whose menarche occurred at age 14 or later.[3-7]

Irregular menstrual cycles during the reproductive years (between menarche and menopause), reflecting abnormal hormonal status, are also a risk factor for current and long-term poor bone health. When the menstrual periods of a young girl become irregular, she not only stops building bone but will also start losing bone that she has already acquired. This situation occurs among some female athletes and frequently among young girls with anorexia nervosa, an eating disorder. The effects of irregular menstrual cycles include a greater risk of stress fractures, scoliosis (curvature of the spine), vertebral compression fractures during the reproductive years, as well as a greater risk of wrist, hip, and vertebral fractures around and after menopause. The therapy for these girls includes restoring normal hormonal levels (through increasing body weight, increasing body fat, or hormone therapy) and adequate amounts of essential nutrients (including calcium, protein, and calories). Even with adequate therapy, the bone loss that occurs during this period may be irreversible.[8-10] See Chapter 6, "The Physical Factors," and Chapter 7, "The Prescription Factors," for more detail.

For women in their reproductive years, another issue affecting hormonal status (and therefore their bone health) is the use of *oral contraceptives.* Although oral contraceptives have been known for decades to be one of the most effective forms of birth control, there has been concern regarding the possible increased risks for blood clots, heart attacks, and stroke. The component of oral contraceptives believed to be primarily responsible for these increased risks is the level of estrogen, and the use of newer, low-estrogen oral contraceptives (containing less than 50 μg) is recommended.[11] A noncontraceptive benefit of oral contraceptive use is a decreased risk for uterine and ovarian cancer; the risk becomes smaller with increasing duration of use.[12-14] In addition, recent research has shown no increased risk of stroke associated with low-estrogen oral contraceptives.[15,16] When used by healthy, nonsmoking women, currently available low-estrogen oral contraceptives are a safe and effective method of birth control.

The most important noncontraceptive benefit of oral contraceptive use during the reproductive years may be their bone-sparing ability to stabilize or even increase bone mass; this positive effect has been reported in studies of both premenopausal and postmenopausal women.[17-25] The positive effect on bone mass is related to the level of hormones used, is proportional to the duration of oral contraceptive use, and is inversely proportional to the age when oral contraceptive use began. In general, the use of oral contraceptives during the reproductive years allows women to enter menopause with a bone density 2-3% higher than that of nonusers—a definite plus in helping to stay out of the critical fracture zone.

Endometriosis is another condition among women in their reproductive years affecting hormonal status and bone health. An estimated 10-20% of women develop this condition, in which tissue lining the uterus (the endometrium) is found outside the uterus or embedded in other tissues of the body, most often the ovaries, Fallopian tubes, or other organs. Although this tissue is outside the uterus, it still responds to the monthly hormonal cycles: swelling in preparation for a fertilized egg, disintegrating when conception does not occur, and sloughing off in preparation for the next cycle. But unlike the normal tissue lining the uterus, this misplaced tissue has no place to escape when it breaks down, and it causes irritation, inflammation, and pain each menstrual cycle. The medical treatment of endometriosis, while reducing the symptoms of this condition, can have an adverse effect on bone health. Gonadotropin-releasing hormone (GnRH) agonists are effective in treating endometritis, but they can result in significant bone loss as early as three months after onset of treatment, and recovery of bone loss may take up to one year after discontinuation of therapy.[26-28] Other medications, such as Danazol, can actually result in bone gain during treatment.[28]

The recurrence rate for endometriosis is estimated to be 5-18% at one year and as high as 40% at five years. When recurrence is diagnosed, additional therapy is necessary. Those medical treatments (such as GnRH agonists) associated with significant bone loss, and with incomplete bone mass recovery before additional treatment is required, result in subsequent bone loss with each treatment, escalating the total bone mass deficit. To alleviate or reduce this adverse effect, some researchers have suggested adding other medications that might counteract this bone loss. In any case, recovery of bone mass after treatment has been shown to be more complete with higher dietary calcium intakes.[26]

Pregnancy

Pregnancy poses a special challenge to a woman's skeleton, when the calcium needs of the growing baby must be met either from her diet or from her own bones. A poor diet during pregnancy can accelerate the loss of calcium from a woman's bones, predisposing her to osteoporosis years later. The hormonal changes that occur during pregnancy increase calcium absorption by the body, and the added weight puts positive stresses on the mother's bones. But if not present in adequate amounts in the mother's diet, calcium will be pulled from her bones to supply the needs of her unborn baby. Pregnancy is an ideal time to reevaluate your diet, for both your sake and the sake of your baby. With today's trends toward postponing pregnancy and toward starting a second family in a woman's thirties or forties, any pregnancy-related bone losses can result in a lower peak bone mass and less bone to lose upon entering menopause.

A woman's diet during pregnancy affects both her own health and the health of her unborn child. During pregnancy, the recommended daily allowances (RDAs) for nearly all nutrients increase, but they do not all double, as might be expected. Only iron, folic acid, and vitamin D increase by 100% or more over nonpregnant levels, whereas calcium and phosphorus increase by 50%; thiamin and vitamin B_6 increase by about 40%; protein, riboflavin, zinc, and vitamin E increase by 20–25%; and selenium, calories, magnesium, iodine, niacin, and vitamins A, B_{12}, C, and K all increase less than 20% (see Table 1).

Building your baby's bones

Calcium has always been a nutrient of special concern during pregnancy. Approximately 30 grams (30,000 mg) of calcium is deposited

TABLE 1

■ ■

Nutrient	Non-pregnant levels	Pregnant levels	Percent increase	Dietary sources
Folic acid	180 μg	400 μg	+122%	Dark green vegetables, citrus fruits
Vitamin D	5 μg	10 μg	+100%	Fortified dairy products
Iron	15 mg	30 mg	+100%	Meats, eggs, breads, cereals, pasta
Calcium	800 mg	1,200 mg	+50%	Milk, cheese, ice cream
Phosphorus	800 mg	1,200 mg	+50%	Meats
Vitamin B_6	1.6 mg	2.2 mg	+38%	Meats, liver, breads, cereals, pasta
Thiamin	1.1 mg	1.5 mg	+36%	Pork, meats, breads, cereals, pasta
Zinc	12 mg	15 mg	+25%	Meats, seafood, eggs
Vitamin E	8 mg	10 mg	+25%	Nuts, oils, enriched grains
Riboflavin	1.3 mg	1.6 mg	+23%	Meats, liver, breads, cereals, pasta
Protein	50 mg	60 mg	+20%	Meats, seafood, poultry, dairy products
Selenium	55 μg	65 μg	+18%	Breads, cereals
Iodine	150 μg	175 μg	+17%	Iodized salt, seafood
Vitamin C	60 mg	70 mg	+17%	Citrus fruits
Energy	2,200 kcal	2,500 kcal	+14%	Proteins, fats, carbohydrates
Magnesium	280 μg	320 μg	+14%	Seafood, beans, breads, cereals, pasta
Niacin	15 mg	17 mg	+13%	Meats, nuts, beans
Vitamin B_{12}	2.0 μg	2.2 μg	+10%	Meats, poultry
Vitamin A	800 μg RE	800 μg RE	No change	Dark green, orange, or yellow produce; liver
Vitamin K	65 μg	65 μg	No change	Green leafy vegetables, dairy products

in the fetal skeleton during pregnancy. The calcium requirement of the baby must be met by the mother with calcium from either her diet or her bones. Although calcium absorption increases by 25–50% during pregnancy, the level of calcium in a woman's diet during pregnancy must still be increased. Calcium is transferred from the mother to the baby at a rate of about 50 mg/day by the middle of pregnancy, increasing to about 330 mg/day by the end of the pregnancy. Changes in calcium metabolism occur early in pregnancy— far in advance of the increased calcium needs of the baby in the last trimester. During the first trimester of pregnancy, additional calcium is deposited in the mother's bones, which is then transferred to the baby later in pregnancy. This drain on the mother's bones is even greater if she is pregnant with multiples (twins, triplets, quadruplets, or more).[29,30] Calcium supplementation during pregnancy has been shown to significantly increase the density of babies' bones. Bone turnover is increased during pregnancy, although with a normal diet, little if any bone mineral is lost.

Prevention of pregnancy complications

Calcium's primary role has been in the prenatal development of teeth and bones, but recent research indicates that this vital nutrient may have another important function as well. Many studies over the past decade with nonpregnant adults have shown that an adequate calcium intake (700–800 mg/day) is protective against **high blood pressure (hypertension),** and that this association is modified by a variety of factors, including diet, lifestyle, and genetics.[31-35] Since 1980, many studies with pregnant women have also found calcium to be related to blood pressure, including **pregnancy-induced hypertension** or **preeclampsia,** as well as to length of gestation.[35-41] Clinical trials with pregnant women given calcium supplements of two grams per day reported that the supplemented groups had significantly lower blood pressure, lower incidence of pregnancy-induced hypertension, and fewer premature births. Although further studies are needed to clarify the relationship between calcium supplementation and the prevention of complications, these results emphasize the importance of adequate calcium intake during pregnancy.

Breast-Feeding

Breast-feeding approximately doubles a woman's daily calcium losses. Since peak bone mass is not achieved for most women until sometime after the childbearing years, bone loss during pregnancy and breast-feeding could potentially have the long-term adverse consequence of increasing a woman's subsequent risk of osteoporosis after menopause. Several studies have shown bone losses of 3–7% do occur during breast-feeding, but that there is an increase in bone mass after weaning.[42-47] The magnitude of bone loss after pregnancy is greater for breast-feeding women than for non–breast-feeding women, but so is the bone gain after weaning. Hormonal status during lactation may alter calcium absorption and utilization at the cellular level. The hormonal changes that accompany breast-feeding, including elevated levels of prolactin and lowered levels of estrogen, progesterone, and testosterone, probably all contribute to excess breakdown even with adequate dietary calcium. Studies have shown that the sooner regular menstrual periods return, the loss of bone with breast-feeding is less, and the gain in bone with weaning is greater.[46] The composition of breast milk is amazingly consistent, regardless of the level of calcium in the woman's diet. As during pregnancy, there can only be two sources for this calcium: either the mother's diet or her bones. Even with a diet adequate in calcium and other essential nutrients, some bone mass is lost during breast-feeding, but hormonal changes at weaning ensure that the loss is replaced. Calcium supplements improve bone health substantially after childbirth for all women and can reduce the amount of bone lost through breast-feeding.[48] Research has shown that with the return of menstruation during weaning, hormone levels also return to prepregnancy levels, resulting in higher mineral absorption and an increase in bone mass. Because of this compensatory gain in bone mass after weaning, breast-feeding has not been shown to be a risk factor for decreased bone mineral density after menopause.

Hysterectomy

For many women, the end of their reproductive years occurs when they undergo a *hysterectomy,* the surgical removal of the uterus. One of the most commonly performed surgical procedures among women (more than 35% of women aged 60–69), hysterectomy is most often done for heavy or painful menstrual bleeding or uterine prolapse. If performed before menopause, the procedure can potentially reduce the blood supply to the ovaries, reducing levels of the bone-sparing hormone estrogen.[49-52] Indirect evidence of this effect has been shown by an increased risk of cardiovascular disease after hysterectomy. Traditionally, the ovaries have been left intact when a hysterectomy is performed because of their positive hormonal effect on skeletal and cardiovascular health. However, many women who have had a hysterectomy, with their ovaries remaining, will develop the classic symptoms of menopause earlier (hot flashes, night sweats, depression) but will be denied hormone replacement therapy because of their age. Declining ovarian function may have caused the menstrual symptoms leading to the hysterectomy; ovarian function declines afterwards in as many as 30% of women.[51] In either situation, it is important to maintain adequate hormone levels before, during, and after menopause to minimize bone loss. More will be said about these issues in Chapter 7, "The Prescription Factors."

Menopause

As with pregnancy, the factors a woman brings with her as she enters menopause have an important influence on her current and future bone health. *Age at menopause* alone is a risk for osteoporosis, with early menopause (under age 45) associated with an increased risk, and later menopause (after age 50) linked with a decreased risk.[53-61] When evaluated together as the *total number of reproductive years* (the time span between menarche and menopause), the association with bone health is even stronger, with an increased risk with less than 30 years, and a decreased risk with more than 40 years.[59-61] Because of the strong link between estrogen and bone health, it's not surprising that the risk for osteoporosis is lowest for women with an early menarche and later menopause—the longest time period of being estrogen-sufficient and potentially achieving the highest peak bone mass. The gender and reproductive issues affecting bone health are summarized in Table 2.

TABLE 2
■■■■■■■■■■■■■■■■■■■■■■■■■■■■■■■■■■■■■■

Risk factor	Increasing risk	Decreasing risk
Gender	Female	Male
Menarche	Late, at age 14 or later	At age 12 or earlier
Menstrual Periods	Irregular	Regular
Menopause	Early, at age 45 or earlier	Later, at age 50 or later
Number of Reproductive Years	30 years or less	40 years or more

As we have discussed risk factors, I'm sure it's becoming increasingly evident why osteoporosis is primarily a woman's disease. In the next chapter we will evaluate the roles of body build, body weight, and body fat in bone health.

CHAPTER 5

The Body Shape Factors

Muscle, Fat, and Body Weight

Bone Basics:

- *One out of six children, one out of five adolescents, and one out of three adults in the United States is overweight.*
- *Four out of ten overweight children and eight out of ten overweight adolescents will become overweight adults.*
- *Women average twice the percent body fat as men.*
- *An ideal percent body fat range for women is 22–26%.*
- *A waist-to-hip ratio for women greater than 0.8 is an increased health risk.*

Why, you ask, is there a chapter on muscle, fat, and body weight in a book about bone health? Simple. These proportions influence your bone health—bone mass is directly related to muscle and inversely related to body fat. In other words, the more muscle and the less fat, the better your bone health.[1] Lifetime weight-bearing exercise is strongly correlated to lean body mass, indicating that low muscle mass, reflecting low levels of physical activity, is a risk factor for low bone mineral density.[2] Diet, exercise, and hormonal status are the key ingredients in achieving and maintaining an ideal weight, appropriate proportions of body muscle and body fat, and good bone health. These same factors are critical in preventing nearly all the chronic diseases and staying in the best health at any age. In this chapter I will discuss how to determine your percent body fat and your ideal body weight for your height.

As I discussed in Chapter 2, "The Age Factor," growth is most rapid during childhood and adolescence. On the average, newborns double their weight by four months and triple their birth weight by one year. From age one to age two, weight increases by about 15 pounds; between the ages of two to six, weight increases by four to six pounds per year. Boys grow the most between the ages of 12 to 16, putting on about 50–60 pounds and about 12 inches in height. By about age 20, most boys are very close to their full adult height. Girls grow the most between the ages of 10 to 14, putting on about 40–50 pounds and about 10 inches in height. Each child grows at a different pace, according to his or her unique genetic blueprint. It is important to keep a balance of good nutrition and adequate physical activity during childhood for good bone development, as well as overall health. Caloric restriction is usually not the answer when children are overweight. Children have the advantage of still growing, and therefore a better tactic is to encourage participation in more physical activity. Better still, join in with your children as a role model, to help them establish healthy eating and physical activity patterns for life.

When it comes to bone health during childhood, height and weight are the most important factors. Physical activity, muscle mass and normal growth, in combination with adequate dietary calcium, are all positively linked with good bone density during childhood and achieving the maximal peak bone mass by young adulthood.[3-8] But according to the most recent national health and nutrition surveys, one out of six children and one out of five adolescents is overweight (see Figures 1 and 2)[9,10] These numbers have been steadily climbing in the United States. Being overweight during childhood is an increased risk for being overweight as an adult.[11] While four out of ten obese 7-year-olds become obese adults, eight out of ten obese adolescents continue to be obese as adults.[12] Although dietary patterns have remained fairly stable among children over several decades, physical activity levels have been declining. Achieving and maintaining an ideal weight for height and physical fitness during childhood are important not only for long-term bone health, but for preventing or reducing the risks for many chronic diseases. For example, heart disease is the number one cause of death in the United States, and we now know that the origins of this chronic disease are in childhood. Both dietary fat intake and body fat during childhood are linked to serum cholesterol levels.[13] In addition, children who are physically fit have healthier levels of all the blood lipids compared to their unfit counterparts—primarily because of lower levels of body fat.[14] Reducing body fat may be important for primary prevention of heart disease in women, beginning in childhood. The Committee on Sports Medicine and Fitness of the American Academy of Pediatrics concludes that low levels of physical activity are the primary factor contributing to the development of obesity among children.[15] The

FIGURE 1
Weight for height percentiles for boys
■ ■

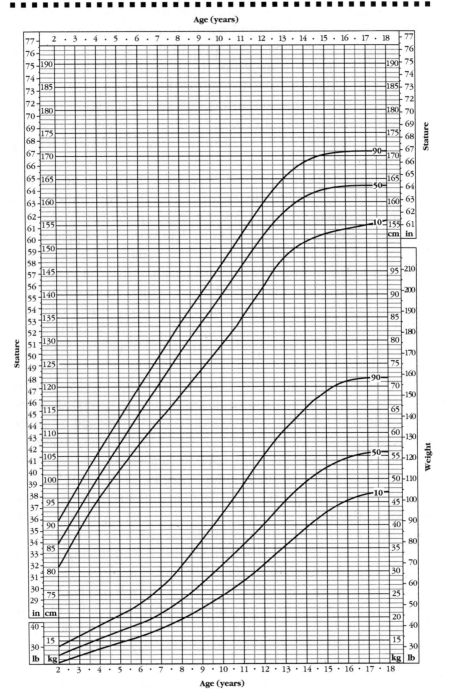

FIGURE 2

Weight for height percentiles for girls

■■■■■■■■■■■■■■■■■■■■■■■■■■■■■■■■■■■■■■■

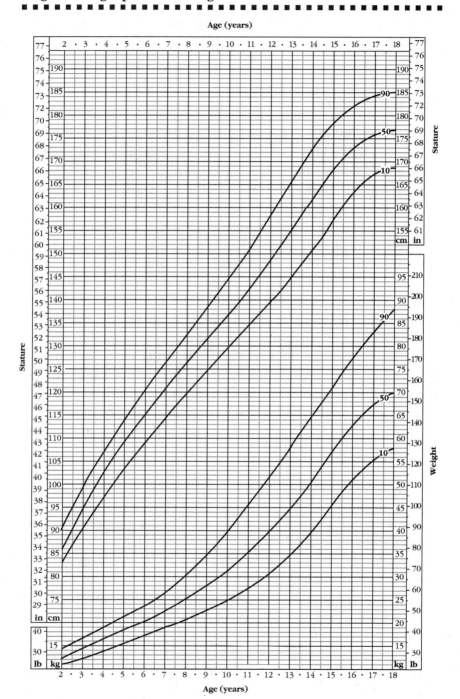

President's Council on Physical Fitness and Sports recommends a minimum of 30 minutes a day of physical activity for students in grades K–12.[16]

Eating Disorders

At the other end of the spectrum is being underweight for height during childhood and adolescence. When extreme, as in the eating disorders of *anorexia nervosa* (self-imposed starvation) and *bulimia* (binging and purging), the effects can retard or reverse bone health. Much more common among girls than boys, individuals with eating disorders have significantly distorted eating attitudes and behaviors as well as emotional problems. They are not voluntarily dieting, and they usually can't discontinue their behavior without professional help. Since eating disorders are primarily a mental disorder, treatment should be centered around mental health services. Eating disorders can delay menarche, the start of regular menstrual periods. As a result of this estrogen deficiency, less bone mass is acquired during the growing years. Even if menstrual function is restored, many of these girls will never achieve the level of bone mass they would have with a normal body weight and age at menarche.[17-19]

From Hourglass to Carafe

An estimated 33 percent of men and 35 percent of women in the United States are overweight, according to the most recent national health and nutrition surveys.[10] For women, this proportion has increased from one out of four in 1960 to more than one out of three in 1991.[20] This increase has occurred among every age group, with one out of five women aged 20–29, one out of three women aged 30-49, and one out of two women aged 50–59 being overweight. As we age, we lose muscle mass and gain body fat—even if our weight is stable.[21-23] This effect is greater for women than for men: at every age, women have twice the percent body fat as men, and for both sexes this percent increases with age. Besides affecting how we fit into our clothes, the amount of fat we carry on our bodies is a central issue for health. Excess weight (as body fat) causes certain diseases and exacerbates others. Being overweight has been linked to heart disease, hypertension (high blood pressure), diabetes, gallbladder disease, and certain types of cancer (such as colon and breast cancer). Those extra pounds can aggravate such conditions as arthritis, back problems, and osteoporosis, as well as increasing the risks of any surgical procedure. Low muscle mass is a risk factor for low bone mineral density, while heavier body weight is protective only when it reflects more muscle.[1,24,25] Without regular physical activity, it's almost impossible to maintain a stable body weight during adulthood.

Why do these changes occur? First, many of us are less physically active than we were when we were younger. Our daily work and responsibilities change, and although we may be even more exhausted at the end of a day at age 40 or 50 than we were at 20 or 30, for most of us it is because of more mental rather than physical demands. Second, as we age, our **basal metabolic rate** slows down—the rate at which we burn calories. For each decade after age 20, our caloric requirements decline by about 2–8 percent, which is why if you continue to eat the same way you did in your twenties when you are in your forties or fifties, you will gain weight each year. Third, because muscle is more metabolically active (burns more calories) than fat, the replacement of muscle by fat as we age lowers our caloric requirements. Although some increase in the proportion of body fat is inevitable with aging, it is possible to limit this increase through diet and exercise. Regular exercise, as discussed in Chapter 6, "The Physical Factors," not only increases the proportion of muscle but will also allow you to eat more liberally. A woman who exercises more like a 25-year-old can eat more like a 25-year-old.

Apples versus Pears

Body shape may be even more important to your health than how much you weigh. In addition to gaining fat and losing muscle with age, the distribution of body fat changes, with most women gaining around the waist. The bigger your waist, the more body fat around your waistline and the greater your risk for many health problems, including cardiovascular disease. Women with "apple" shapes, who carry most of their fat in the torso—as abdominal or waistline fat—tend to have more health problems than "pears," women who carry their weight below the waistline. Women who smoke tend to have more waistline fat, which in turn is linked to an increased risk for heart disease. Hormones play a big role in how body fat is distributed. Because estrogens tend to increase body fat below the waist and androgens (male hormones) tend to put it on around the waist, the hormonal changes around menopause favor putting on waistline fat.

Bathroom Scales and Tape Measures

The number on the bathroom scale tells only part of the story, depending on your height, age, and level of physical activity. Two other measures will help you determine your percent body fat and whether or not your weight-for-height is within an optimal range: your body mass index (BMI) and your hip measurement. Your BMI is a measure of your weight adjusted for your height. To calculate your BMI, multiple your weight (in pounds) times 700, then divide that number by your height (in inches) squared. For example, if you are 5'4" and weigh 140 pounds, your BMI is 24.8. The normal weight-for-height BMI range is 19.8–26.0. Ideally, women should have about 22–26 percent body fat, but the average woman has about 32 percent or more. Gymnasts average about 14 percent body fat, aerobic instructors about 17 percent, and swimmers about 20 percent.

In Table 1, according to your height, I've listed the normal weight ranges for women with a medium build, the range of hip measurements corresponding to 22–26 percent body fat, and the BMIs for the weight range for each height. If your hip measurements are higher than these ranges for your height, then your percent body fat is probably higher than this ideal range, too.

So, the take-home message is to:

- *Keep your BMI within the ideal range for your height.*
- *Keep your body weight stable.*

- *Keep your percent body fat within an ideal range.*
- *Keep your muscle and lose your fat.*

How can you achieve these goals? Diet and exercise—the key ingredients in nearly every health maintenance program—can help keep your body weight from inching higher every year.[26] In the next chapter I will discuss physical activity and how to integrate it into your daily life, and in Chapters 9 and 10 I will address the issue of food.

TABLE 1

▪▪

Height	Weight* Medium build**	Hip measurement, 22–26% body fat	Body mass index***
4'10"	108–120 lbs	30–32.5"	22.5–25.0
4'11"	110–123 lbs	31–33.5"	22.1–24.7
5'	112–126 lbs	31.5–34"	21.8–24.5
5'1"	116–129 lbs	32–34.5"	21.8–24.3
5'2"	118–132 lbs	32.5–35"	21.5–24
5'3"	121–135 lbs	33.5–36"	21.3–23.8
5'4"	124–138 lbs	34–36.5"	21.2–23.6
5'5"	127–141 lbs	34.5–37"	21–23.4
5'6"	130–144 lbs	35.5–38"	20.9–23.1
5'7"	133–147 lbs	36–38.5"	20.7–22.9
5'8"	136–150 lbs	36.5–39.5"	20.6–22.7
5'9"	139–153 lbs	37.5–40"	20.4–22.5
5'10"	142–156 lbs	38–40.5"	20.3–22.3
5'11"	145–159 lbs	38.5–41"	20.1–22.1
6'	148–162 lbs	39.5–42"	20.1–21.9

*1983 Metropolitan Life Insurance Company figures.

**10% lower for small body build, 10% higher for large body build.

CHAPTER 6

The Physical Factors

Exercise and Physical Activity

Bone Basics:

- *On bedrest, as much bone is lost in two weeks as would otherwise have been lost in two years.*
- *Athletic amenorrhea may result in a permanent bone deficit.*
- *Bones must act against resistance to grow stronger.*
- *Physically active children emerge from adolescence with 5–10% more bone mass.*
- *One out of three adults do not participate in any leisure-time physical activity.*
- *Regular exercise should include a combination of endurance and strength training.*

A common sight in the Swedish countryside are white-haired grandmothers riding three-wheeled bicycles equipped with large baskets—obviously doing the grocery shopping or other chores. In Amsterdam, during the morning and evening rush hours, thousands of bicycles fill the streets and narrow bridges, and cars are clearly in the minority. College students, retirees, businessmen and -women, and mothers and fathers with their grade-school children on the bicycle back seats are typical of the commuters in the Netherlands. The physical activity that is such an integral part of everyday life in these countries is a major factor in their substantially lower national rates of osteoporosis compared to the United States, where we generally have a more sedentary lifestyle. Even in areas like Hong Kong, where there is a genetic predisposition to decreased bone mass, the incidence of osteoporosis is low and most adults have healthy bones because of the compensating effect of high physical activity.[1] But the bone health of even the active Europeans has declined compared to their ancestors—primarily due to less physical activity in their lives today than generations ago.[2]

Remember Chapter 1, when I talked about bone modeling and remodeling? Well, physical activity and the forces we impose on our bones are critical factors in making our bones rebuild and remodel. Unlike a nonliving structure, which is weakened by physical forces over time, our skeletons are alive and growing, responding to mechanical stress by increasing in both mass and density. Weight-bearing exercise, such as biking, baseball, basketball, soccer, skating, tennis, weightlifting, aerobics, dancing, and walking, improves your bone health in several ways. First, this type of exercise stimulates bone formation by making your bones work against resistance. Second, it improves your muscle strength, which in turn pulls and tugs on your bones. Third, exercise improves your balance and coordination, reducing your risk of falls and accidents, which are more likely to lead to fractures if your bones are weak. Weight-bearing exercise can improve your bone health at any age, and although the effect is influenced by all of your other risk factors, the most important one is your age. Physical activity may have the greatest effect during childhood, with active children emerging from adolescence with 5–10% greater bone mass.[3] This advantage may help in attaining a greater peak bone mass in adulthood. In addition, regular participation in sports during childhood and adolescence increases the likelihood of being more physically active later in life.[4] Taken together, the cumulative effect of lifetime physical activity is significantly associated with the best bone health at every age.[5-7] In this chapter we are going to look at the spectrum of physical activity and its effect on bone health, how physical activity influences our bones at different ages, and determine the best exercise for you right now. Let's get moving!

Form Follows Function

Bone health requires the right balance of hormones, nutrition, and exercise—a picture I'm sure you are beginning to piece together as you read through this book. A deficiency in one component can't be made up for by doubling up on another—it doesn't work that way. Without this balance, bone health suffers. The two extremes of this balance are complete physical inactivity—absolute bedrest—and the intense physical training of elite athletes. Bedrest, which we traditionally associate with being beneficial to health, is actually one of the worst things you can do to your bones. Physicians have long observed that patients on bedrest lost bone mass, as evidenced from X-rays. But what is surprising is just how fast this happens, even among individuals who are otherwise healthy. Complete bedrest results in the loss of as much bone mass in two weeks as would otherwise have been lost in two years! The trend in medicine today is to get patients up as quickly as possible after an illness or surgery, and we now know that, in addition to bone loss, immobility actually slows the healing process. If you do need to be confined to bed for any length of time, getting out of bed at least once a day for 30 minutes or so, if possible, may prevent significant bone loss.

At the other end of the physical activity spectrum are world-class athletes. If there is a strong link between physical activity and bone health, you would expect these individuals to have the largest bone mass and the greatest bone density, and that's exactly what most studies have found. But bone health suffers, even among these individuals, when the balance is disrupted among those three important key ingredients: hormones, nutrition, and exercise. As discussed in Chapters 4 and 5, high levels of physical activity, often combined with strict dieting to maintain a lean physique, can delay menarche in adolescents or cause menstrual cycles to become irregular or cease completely among girls and women who had been menstruating regularly. This disturbance of normal hormonal levels, particularly estrogen, results in a rapid loss of bone mass, despite the vigorous regimen of physical activity. Termed the "female athlete triad,"[8,9] this combination of factors can result in failure to achieve adequate bone mass during the growing years or premature loss of bone mass already attained, and ultimately a lower peak bone mass. All adolescent and some adult athletes are potentially at risk, particularly those who participate in appearance-based and endurance sports and those who compete at an elite level.

Delayed menarche (when menstruation begins after age 16) is frequent among ballet dancers and gymnasts—two activities where girls begin strenuous training as early as five or six years of age. This disruption in the normal hormonal environment at the critical time of the adolescent growth spurt can have several adverse consequences, including the development of *scoliosis* (curvature of the spine) and *stress fractures.* [10-13] Athletes who experience irregular menstrual cycles or secondary amenorrhea (the absence of menstrual periods for three or more consecutive months) have significantly lower bone mineral density and less bone mass compared to those who menstruate regularly.[10,11,13,14-21] Even with a return of regular menstrual cycles, decreased physical activity, and an adequate or even calcium-supplemented diet, the bone mass that was lost may never be completely recovered.[22-24] This effect has raised concern among bone researchers that *athletic amenorrhea,* particularly among adolescents, may result in a permanent bone deficit that may not be recovered during later adulthood.

Vigorous training may also adversely affect hormone levels (and therefore bone health) in young men as well. One study showed that, compared to male rowers and sedentary controls, male triathletes had lower serum testosterone levels.[25] Another study reported that, compared to sedentary male adolescents of the same age, cyclists who had trained an average of 10 hours per week during the prior two years had significantly lower bone mass and bone density.[26] Although poor bone health is less common among males, a disturbance in the balance between those three key ingredients—hormones, nutrition, and exercise—can have the same adverse effects on their skeletons, particularly during the adolescent growth spurt.

Anna is a ballerina. She began dancing at the age of eight years and joined a professional troupe at the age of 16. She is 5'8" tall and weighs 100 pounds. At age 18, her height is at the 95th percentile for her age and her weight is at the 25th percentile. Her monthly periods have not begun yet. Over the past year she has suffered several stress fractures in her toes, and last month she fractured her wrist when she fell during practice.

Carrie is a gymnast. She has been on her local team since age 10, and by age 12 she had made it to the state championships. At age 13 she sprained her ankle during practice and took a month off from training. During that month her weight increased from 85 pounds to 100 pounds (from the 10th percentile to the 50th percentile), and her monthly periods began.

Both of these girls illustrate how extremes in exercise and low body fat can delay the onset of menarche. If we measured their bone density, we would probably find changes leading to osteoporosis. The lack of estrogen causes the release of calcium already stored within the bones, quickly making them thin and fragile. Evidence of this can already be seen for Anna, who at age 18 has not yet experienced menarche and has already had several stress fractures. In addition to being more susceptible to fractures, once they occur healing is much slower in the absence of adequate estrogen. For Carrie, her vigorous physical activity, low body fat, and delayed menarche during early adolescence probably resulted in less bone growth, in length, mass, and density, than should have occurred. Compared to running, which transmits a force (also known as *impact load*) to the spine of 3–5 times the body weight with each step, components of gymnastic routines, such as dismounting from the parallel bars, transmit impact loads equal to 15–20 times the body weight. Research suggests that the stress of repetitive compression so common in gymnastics may injure the epiphyseal plates (the area of bone still growing in length), ultimately resulting in less growth of the legs.[27-29] Carrie's weight gain during convalescence was enough to trigger the hormonal changes initiating menarche. With regular menstrual periods, Carrie's bone health should improve, but if she loses weight again, her periods will probably stop and her bone health will suffer once again.

But with the right balance of hormones, nutrition, and exercise, bones get stronger and stronger—this has been demonstrated in studies of all types of physical activity. To strengthen bones, they must work against resistance, and this positive effect is very site-specific. For example, the average figure skater has significantly greater bone density in her pelvis and legs but no differences in bone structure in her spine or arms.[30] Weight lifters have greater bone densities in the spine and legs, and this increase varies with duration: older weight lifters have even stronger bones than their younger counterparts.[31,32]

An even clearer example of the effect of physical activity on bone health comes from squash and tennis players. Not only is bone mineral density and content greater in the stroke arm (by as much as one-third), but that arm may also be significantly longer.[33-35] The repetitive resistance (volleying the ball) during growth is believed to be responsible for the unique bone changes among these athletes, particularly when strenuous training began before or during puberty.

Bones must act against resistance to grow stronger. Resistance can be in the form of working *against gravity* (such as standing or walking), *against additional body weight* (running, jumping, or dancing), or *against a force* (tennis, squash, racquetball, baseball) or *weights* (free weights or weight machines) (see Figure 1). In activities such as biking, the bones in the legs are acting against resistance, while the spine works only against gravity. Even less work against resistance occurs with swimming, because of the buoyancy of the water. This type of force, known as an *active*

FIGURE 1

Work against gravity (standing/walking); against additional body weight (running/jumping/dancing); against a force (tennis/baseball); against weights (free weights/weight machines)
■■

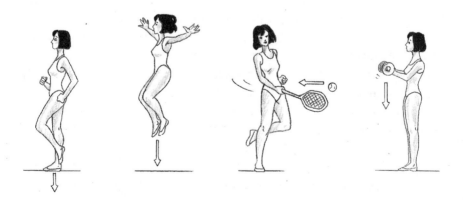

load, acts on bones primarily through muscle contraction. Although members of college-level swimming teams have substantial muscle strength, they have lower bone mass than other athletes or even sedentary individuals of the same age.[36] In studies of children before and during puberty, those involved in weight-bearing sports had significantly greater femoral and spinal bone densities compared to those involved in competitive swimming.[37] So, while swimming provides a wonderful cardiovascular, low-impact workout, unfortunately it does little for your bones.

So, I hope you are beginning to understand how exercise is a positive factor affecting bone health—as long as we keep in mind the need to work against resistance as well as the other key factors of nutrition and hormone status. As I have mentioned many times before, age is the most important factor when it comes to our bones; with physical activity, age again is a key ingredient. Physical activity at younger ages, when the growth rate of bones is naturally at its greatest level, appears to be more important for the development of maximal peak bone mass and to be essential in maintaining bone mass later in life.[3,5,38-43] In contrast to bone changes during later years, at younger ages the skeleton may be more responsive to the effects of exercise because mineral is acquired on both the periosteal and endosteal surfaces of bone. The other important factors positively related to bone mineral density and content are *number of years of participation or training and muscle strength.* The results of the Amsterdam Growth and Health Study, a 15-year longitudinal study of males and females from age 13 to age 28, suggest that regular weight-bearing exercise and at least a normal age-related body weight during adolescence and young adulthood are of key importance in reaching the highest peak bone mass by the end of the third decade.[40] In another study of college-aged women, both past and present levels of exercise as well as lean body mass were factors most strongly linked to bone health.[44] In this study, both past and present levels of dietary calcium and menstrual status were also significant factors, but to a much lesser effect.

We know physical activity is good for us—not just for bone health. Regular exercise helps reduce the risks for heart disease, diabetes, colon cancer, hypertension, depression, and obesity, just to name a few. An estimated 250,000 deaths in the United States each year (12% of total deaths) are attributable to a lack of regular exercise.[45,46] Yet one-third or more of all adults have no leisure-time physical activity, and this proportion increases with age, is higher among women compared to men, and is more common in winter than in summer months.[47] So what's the solution? To integrate physical activity into our daily lives, as part of healthy habits, and as role models for our children and peers. Remember, exercise during the growing years may be important for achieving greater peak bone mass, as well as reducing the risk of heart disease in later life.[48]

Get Out and Move

Lack of time is the most commonly cited barrier to participating in physical activity, and injury is a frequent reason for stopping regular exercise. If you're like me, you put in a long day at work, and the last thing you want to do when you get home is exercise. It's easy to talk yourself out of it during the ride home—"I'm so tired, I barely have enough energy to make dinner and listen to the evening news"—right? Well, the best advice I've heard yet came from my friend Loretta, a marathon runner, who is 50+ but has the physique of a 22-year-old. Loretta, who runs several miles every day, suggested to me that the hardest part is getting into the exercise clothes. "Once you have your exercise clothes on, those sneakers tied up, you're going to do it—you're going to exercise—no doubt about it." And she's right. I began a program of regular exercise about a year ago, and I go so far as to lay out clean exercise clothes on the bed when I leave for work in the morning (when I'm bright-eyed and ready for the day, and optimistic about exercising that evening). Loretta also advises that it's important not to get distracted by anything once you get home—don't open the mail, listen to your phone messages, start a load of laundry. All of these things can wait that hour or so it takes you to exercise.

And you will be so glad you did. The seemingly paradoxical fact about exercise is that you feel energized after a good workout—you are limber, glowing, awake, and alert, all the things you weren't before you started, when you were mentally talking yourself out of going to the gym! So try to remember that wonderful feeling the next time you begin to slip back into your old "couch potato" ways. Exercise is the best tonic around, with more health benefits than any other therapy I know!

But you don't have to go to a gym to exercise. Better yet, integrate physical activity into your daily life. In my younger days I ran a nutrition clinic on the fifth floor of the outpatient building at the Columbia-Presbyterian Medical Center in New York City. Besides a daily regimen of swimming (I had been the only girl on an all-boys team back in high school in the 1960s), I made it a habit of always walking up the stairs at work and taking the elevator down. Of course, I was in much more of a rush about everything when I was in my twenties so I ended up walking downstairs, too. But stairs are only one example. If you take public transportation or a car to work, consider getting off a few blocks earlier and walking the rest of the way, and steadily increasing the distance with each week (weather permitting). At lunchtime, take a walk or, better yet, do some chores so that you will have more time to yourself after work. Take advantage of the seasons—raking the leaves or building a snowman are also forms of exercise.

How Much Exercise Is Enough?

No matter how old (or young) you are, regardless of your medical condition or level of fitness, everyone can benefit from a program of regular physical activity. But how much is enough? To be the most effective, experts recommend *30 minutes or more of moderate-level physical activity on most days of the week.*[49] Moderate-level physical activity includes walking briskly (at a rate of 3–4 miles per hour), cycling (under 10 miles per hour), swimming (with moderate effort), general calisthenics, golf (either pulling the golf cart or carrying the clubs), canoeing, mowing the lawn, raking leaves, house painting, house cleaning, or house repairing. At this level and duration of activity, which expends about 200 calories per day, you should expect to see and feel substantial health benefits in as quickly as a few weeks. This 30-minutes-a-day prescription can also be accumulated with shorter periods of activity: walking up stairs, walking instead of driving, pedaling a stationary bike while watching the evening news. If performed at an intensity equivalent to brisk walking, such activities as gardening, housework, dancing, and playing with children can all contribute to your daily total. Of course, working up to longer periods of increasing exertion will result in greater benefits. The key message, though, is to get started. A common mistake is to begin too ambitiously, get discouraged and quit. Don't set your immediate goals too high, or you probably won't keep up your routine.

How Do You Measure Exercise Intensity?

Simple. Your heart rate will tell you. Your **target heart rate** during moderate physical activity should be between 60 and 90% of your **ideal maximum heart rate.** To calculate your ideal maximum heart rate, subtract your age from 220; your target heart rate should be between 60 and 90 percent of this number. For example, if you are 45 years old, your ideal maximum heart rate is 175 beats per minute; your target heart rate would be between 60 and 90 percent of 175, or 105 and 158 beats per minute. During physical activity or exercise, check your heart rate by taking your pulse at your wrist. Your pulse for 15 seconds (one-fourth of a minute) should be between 26 and 40 beats. If your pulse is lower than this range, pick up your pace; if it's above this range, slow down a bit.

High- versus Low-Impact Activities

If it sounds like I'm keen on walking—well, I am. It's the most benign kind of physical activity, good for all ages and levels of fitness. Walking has been shown to improve bone health, even among older adults, particularly when combined with a resistance or strength routine. It's also been shown to be therapeutic in slowing the rate of bone loss among older men and women. The best bone health is achieved when the physical activity regimen includes both endurance and strength training, movement against resistance or weight. For sedentary individuals, and even elderly adults, walking or low-impact or water aerobics are the best type of exercises to start. High-impact physical activities include running and jogging, gymnastics, basketball, volleyball, aerobics, dancing, downhill skiing, and rope skipping. Low-impact physical activities include walking and hiking, cycling (including stationary cycling), swimming, rowing, cross-country skiing, golf, gardening, and housework. The American Heart Association recommends that for individuals older than age 40, special precautions be taken if participating in high-impact activities.[50] These precautions include (1) initiating the activity at low levels and increasing slowly; (2) allowing a day of rest between exercise periods to permit gradual adaptation to stress and strains; and (3) paying more attention to warm-up and cool-down periods with stretches.

Strength as Well as Endurance

Another important reason to exercise regularly is to improve and maintain your overall strength. Walking benefits your spine, hips, and legs, but your hands, wrists, arms, and shoulders need a workout, too. As discussed in Chapter 5, "The Body Shape Factors," we lose muscle mass as we age, and if we don't continue to stimulate our muscles, we lose strength. Besides looking and feeling better, it's great to have the ability to carry those groceries, lift those boxes, close that minivan door—and remember, strong bones are inside strong muscles. I first started strength training several years ago, shortly after I took up scuba diving. My main motivation for increasing my strength was to be able to carry around all that scuba gear; it doesn't weigh much when you have it on in the water, but carrying around 40–50 pounds of wet suit, fins, and air tank on land was a reality check on how much muscle strength I had lost during my thirties and early forties.

Free weights or weight machines are a good choice to build and maintain muscle strength, with the goal of progressing to heavier weights and more repetitions. To avoid injury and to assure that you are performing the routines correctly, you should begin any new program under the guidance of a physical therapist or professional trainer; your primary care physician can give you a referral to these specialists in exercise and physical activity. In the Appendix I've listed several of my favorite exercise magazines; they have regular columns featuring exercises for specific muscle groups, as well as inspirational stories about real people and their physical activity programs. To get you started, I've outlined below my routine for building strength and flexibility. I'm a busy woman, and I designed this routine to get the most out of the fewest exercises and in the least amount of time. Remember, start slow, maintain good body alignment, and use light weights and few repetitions. As the routines become easier, add more weight and repetitions. You will soon see the difference in your ability to do daily activities like carrying groceries, moving furniture, or carrying books.

Barbara's Exercise Routine:

My routine takes about one hour to complete, and I do it three-four times a week. On other days, I walk during my lunch hour, and I make it a regular habit to take the stairs instead of the elevator. My routine includes a combination of endurance and strength training, and gives me a complete body workout. For endurance, I spend 20 minutes on the **treadmill**, *walking at 4 miles per hour and jogging at 5 miles per hour. Right now I spend more time walking than jogging, but my goal is to spend most or all of the time jogging. Next, I spend 20 minutes on the* **StairMaster**. *Last, I end my exercise session with free weights and the weight machines.*

With free weights, I do three exercises, each with a different focus.

- *First, using 2-5 pound weights, I do* **reverse wrist curls**, *three sets of 15 repetitions (see Figure 2). This exercise works the flexor and extensor muscles of the forearms and wrists, improving strength and flexibility. Like many of*

FIGURE 2
Reverse wrist curls
▪▪

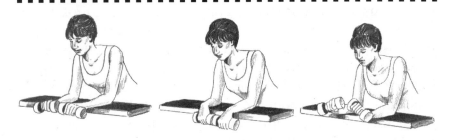

you, I spend hours a day at the computer keyboard, and I find that this set of exercises helps reduce symptoms of carpal tunnel syndrome.

- *Second, using 10-pound weights, I do **bench presses**, three sets of ten repetitions (see Figure 3). This exercise works the muscles of the chest, the shoulders, and the back of the upper arms (triceps)—an area that is a trouble spot for many women, including me. As you do this exercise, resist arching your back. By turning your hands inward, you work the muscles of the upper chest, whereas turning your hands forward works the muscles of the mid-chest.*

- *Third, using a single 10-pound weight, I do **pullovers**, three sets of 10 repetitions (see Figure 4). This exercise works the lower portion of the chest as well as the backs of the upper arms.*

The last part of my routine includes working out on the weight machines. The advantage of exercising on this type of equipment is that it's easier to maintain good body alignment, and each machine is specifically designed to work a certain set of muscles. With weight machines I do three exercises—again, each with a different focus.

- *First, using 50 pounds of weight, I do **lat pull-downs**, four sets of ten repetitions (see Figure 5). This exercise strengthens and tones the muscles of both the upper and*

FIGURE 3
Bench press with free weights
■■■

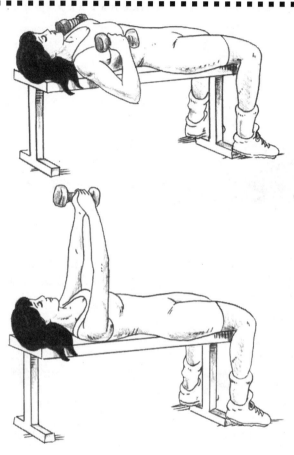

FIGURE 4
Pullover with a single weight

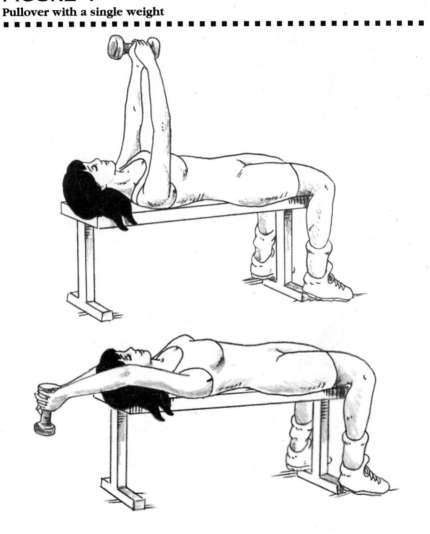

FIGURE 5

Lat pull-downs, with wide and narrow grips

▪▪

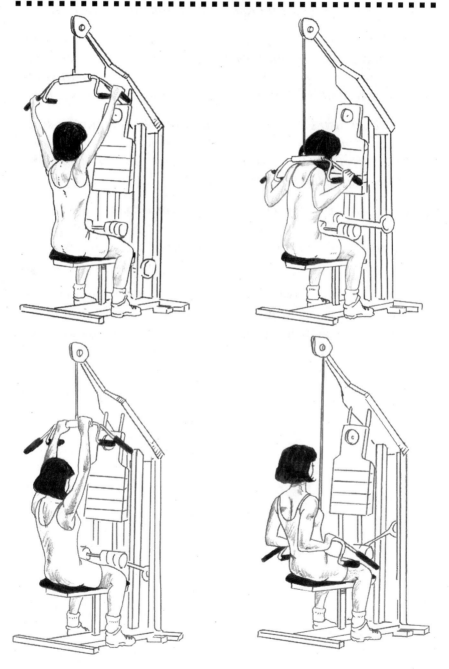

lower back, helping to support the spine. I alternate sets using a wide grip and a narrow grip, which fully works both the upper and lower latissimus dorsi muscles.

• *Second, using 50 pounds of weight, I do **leg extensions** using a **leg extension machine,** three sets of ten repetitions (see Figure 6). This exercise works the mid and lower portion of the fronts of the thighs: the quadriceps muscles.*

• *Third, using 50 pounds of weight, I do **leg curls** using a **leg curl machine,** three sets of ten repetitions (see Figure 7). This exercise works the mid and lower portion of the backs of the thighs: the hamstring muscles.*

*I also do two other exercises, **leg extensions** (see Figure 8) to firm the muscles of the abdomen, and **push-ups** (see Figure 9) to firm the upper arms. All of these exercises work the muscles and associated joints, so you get a dual benefit.*

The ultimate goal to keep in mind when it comes to physical activity and bone health is to *get started and keep moving*— begin and maintain a program of regular physical activity that suits you and your lifestyle. Let's get moving!

FIGURE 6
Leg extensions with leg extension machine
▪▪▪▪▪▪▪▪▪▪▪▪▪▪▪▪▪▪▪▪▪▪▪▪▪▪▪▪▪▪▪▪▪▪▪▪▪

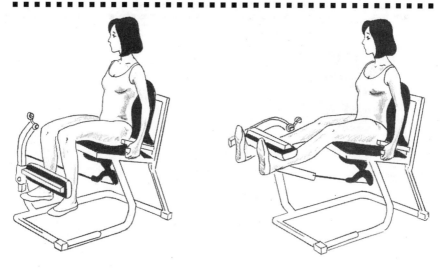

FIGURE 7
Leg curls with a leg curl machine
▪▪▪▪▪▪▪▪▪▪▪▪▪▪▪▪▪▪▪▪▪▪▪▪▪▪▪▪▪▪▪▪▪▪▪▪▪

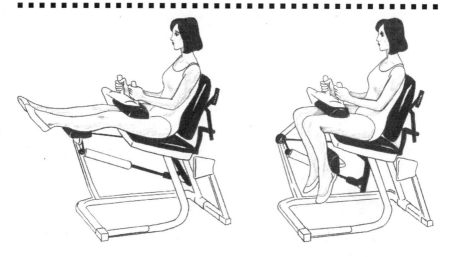

FIGURE 8
Leg extensions (ballet exercise, for stomach muscles)
■■

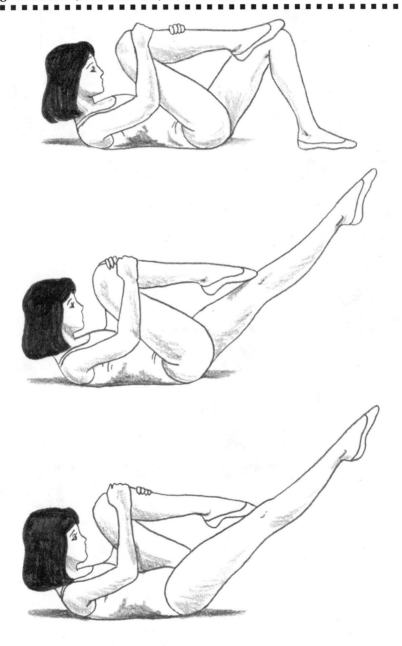

FIGURE 9
Push-ups

▪▪▪▪▪▪▪▪▪▪▪▪▪▪▪▪▪▪▪▪▪▪▪▪▪▪▪▪▪▪▪▪▪

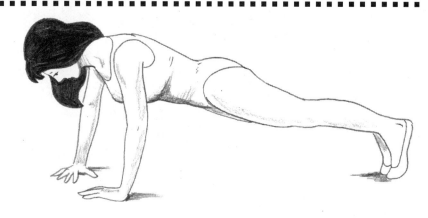

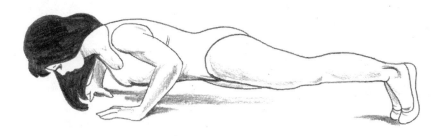

CHAPTER 7

The Prescription Factor

Hormones, Medications, and Supplements

Bone Basics:

- *During menopause, total bone mass is reduced by about 15%.*

- *Women lose more than 25% of their peak bone mass by age 60, and 50% by age 70.*

- *Between ages 50 and 94, a woman's risk of death from heart disease is 10-fold greater than her risk of death from breast cancer.*

- *Hormone replacement therapy (HRT) can reduce the risks for both hip fractures and heart disease by 50%.*

- *HRT reduces a woman's risk of colon cancer, improves the symptoms of menopause, mental abilities, and skin changes, but may increase the risk for breast and uterine cancer.*

In this chapter I am going to discuss three groups of medications that can affect bone health: hormones, prescription medications, and calcium supplements. Hormones and hormone replacement therapy (HRT) are issues that are always in the news—millions of women have used hormones as oral contraceptives during their childbearing years, and most women know that HRT is a decision they must face in their forties or fifties. In this chapter I'll tell you about HRT, the risks and benefits, and how to balance both to make your own choice. I'll also discuss other bone-building medications currently available and those still in the experimental stage. Other prescription medications can also influence your bone health, and I will discuss them, too. Last, I will present information about calcium supplements—how to choose the best ones and how to take them to improve their effectiveness. Let's begin.

Hormones are chemical compounds that cause specific effects in targeted cells and tissues in the body. They are essential, powerful factors affecting bone health, with low levels or deficiencies greatly increasing the susceptibility of bones to osteoporosis. For example, a deficiency of calcitriol, the active form of vitamin D, can dramatically reduce intestinal absorption of calcium, while low levels of estrogen drain calcium from the bones at an alarming rate. Three main groups of hormones influence bone health: the *calcium-regulating hormones* (parathyroid hormone, vitamin D, and calcitonin), the *growth-regulating hormones* (growth hormone, glucocorticoids, thyroid hormone, and insulin), and the *sex hormones* (estrogen, prolactin, progestins, and testosterone). Low levels or deficiencies of any one of these hormones at any stage in the life cycle can lead to changes in bone development and an increased risk for osteoporosis.

The Advantages of HRT

Of all of these hormones, estrogen is one of the most important ones for women. This hormone is a critical player in the transformation of girls into young women during adolescence, in the monthly menstrual cycle, and (because of declining levels) in the rapid bone loss experienced by postmenopausal women. Without the protective effects of estrogen, we lose between 2 and 10% of our bone mass *every year* during the first years after menopause. Estrogen replacement therapy (also known as hormone replacement therapy, or HRT, when combined with another hormone, progesterone) is intended to mimic the body's natural hormone cycle that occurred before menopause. This replacement both relieves the commonly experienced symptoms of menopause (hot flashes, depression and mood swings, vaginal dryness) and protects from the accelerated loss of bone mass. Because of the increased risk of uterine cancer among women who used estrogen alone, progestin (the synthetic form of the hormone progesterone) was added to reduce or eliminate this side effect. The usual oral dosage during menopause—0.625 mg of conjugated estrogens (a combination of naturally occurring estrogens) plus 2.5 mg of the progestin medroxyprogesterone acetate every day or other regimen in a cyclic fashion as prescribed by a physician—is about one-sixth the dosage used in birth control pills. The bone-sparing effects of estrogen are dependent on the dose but not on the route (pills, patches, or creams) or the addition of progestin.

To understand how HRT works after menopause, let's back-track for a minute and look at estrogen's natural role in a woman's body. Receptors for this hormone are found in more than 300 different tissues, ranging from brain to bone, from breasts to skin. All these sites respond to the presence (and absence or deficiency) of estrogen. During puberty, rising levels of estrogen and other hormones produced by the ovaries trigger the changes that transform girls into women. At menopause, essentially the reverse of this process occurs. Estrogen levels begin to decline during our thirties, although the effects are barely noticeable. By our forties, the effects are more obvious, with a fall in fertility, skin and hair changes, more mood swings, and often a decline in our sexual drive (the libido). During this transitional period, known as the *perimenopause,* hormone levels can fluctuate erratically, resulting in the classic symptoms of menopause: hot flashes, heart palpitations, night sweats, mood swings, headaches, depression, irregular periods, and vaginal dryness. Nearly nine out of ten women experience some of these symptoms, often lasting as long as five years if untreated. For most women, symptoms disappear within one year after their last period (the definition of menopause). Although the average age at menopause is 51, many women begin to experience symptoms in their late forties. For a woman who has undergone surgical removal of her uterus and ovaries (hysterectomy and oophorectomy), menopause occurs abruptly. HRT can greatly relieve these *perimenopause* symptoms, as well as preserving bone health, but not every woman is a candidate for these medications.[1] HRT is contraindicated for women with a personal history of breast, ovarian, or uterine cancer, fibroids, liver disease, or problems with blood clotting. In uterine cancer, however, estrogen replacement therapy can be reinstituted after a certain time period has elapsed since the cancer treatment.

HRT is effective only if taken long-term, probably for life. Research has demonstrated this benefit with the prevention of heart disease, the number one killer of women in the United States.[2] Estrogen helps to keep the levels of low-density lipoprotein cholesterol (LDL, the "bad" cholesterol) low and the high-density lipoprotein cholesterol (HDL, the "good" cholesterol) high.[3-5] Estrogen also acts directly on blood vessels, causing them to dilate and improve blood flow. These effects help explain why premenopausal women have much less heart disease than men. Without HRT, within a decade or so after menopause, men and women have nearly identical risks for heart attack. For women over age 50, cardiovascular disease is the number one cause of death. Much of a woman's greater life expectancy can be attributed to estrogen's protective effect. Some investigators believe that HRT has a beneficial protective effect against the development of Alzheimer's disease.

The key issue for bone health is the sharp decline in estrogen levels around menopause, which results in a rapid depletion of bone mass by about 15% overall, although this decline levels off within about five years. As discussed in Chapter Two, "The Age Factor," most women achieve their peak bone mass, the maximum amount of bone present before age-related losses begin, well before their 40th birthday. After about age 40, women begin to slowly lose bone mass at the rate of about 1% per year in part because of declining levels of the bone-sparing hormone estrogen. Within the first 5-7 years after menopause, we can lose as much as 2-8% of vertebral (spinal) bone and as much as 20% of femoral (hip joint) bone. Without HRT, most women will have lost more than 25% of their peak bone mass by age 60, and 50% by age 70. Although the rate of bone loss slows after age 60, the bone that is remodeled is structurally less dense and less sturdy.

The World Health Organization defines osteoporosis as a bone mass two standard deviations below the mean for normal, healthy young adults—in other words, a bone mass falling below the normal range.[6] For each reduction in bone mass of one standard deviation, the risk of fracture doubles.[7] The rapid menopausal bone loss results in an overall decline in bone mass by about 15%, equivalent to one standard deviation from the mean for normal adults.[8] For women with a peak bone mass already one standard deviation below the mean, the bone loss experienced during menopause (equivalent to a drop of an additional standard deviation) can quickly put her in the critical fracture zone—at high risk of developing fractures. Peak bone mass and estrogen levels are critical factors in determining postmenopausal bone health and fracture risk. Long-term HRT improves calcium absorption by the digestive system, improves conservation of calcium by the kidneys, and prevents osteoporosis in 8 out of 10 women. HRT is believed by many researchers to be central in maintaining bone health after menopause, with maximal benefit effect when initiated in the menopausal period and continued into late life.[9,10] In combination with exercise and diet, hormones are one of the three key ingredients to building and keeping good bones at every age.

The Risks of HRT

The major drawback with long-term HRT is the increased risk for certain cancers. When estrogen was originally prescribed alone, the risk for uterine cancer was much greater.[11] Today it is prescribed in lower dosages and in combination with the hormone progestin, which inhibits the growth of the uterine lining. Only a woman who has had her uterus removed (hysterectomy) can safely take estrogen alone. Even on combination therapy, it is important to monitor for uterine cancer if you have any abnormal bleeding. Current evidence suggests a slight, if any, increased possibility of developing breast cancer with long-term HRT.[12-14] Most studies report that this increase occurs after 10–15 years of estrogen use and that both the type and dosage of estrogen may be at fault. We still don't know the effect of combination therapy on a woman's risk of breast cancer, and studies that are currently under way should provide us with answers within a few years.

Another risk of HRT is the development of gallbladder disease. For women who are at risk of developing gallbladder attacks, oral HRT should be avoided because it increases the formation of cholesterol crystals in the bile ducts, increasing the risk of the formation of gallstones.

To put these risks in perspective, between the ages of 50 and 94, a woman's risk of death from heart disease is more than 10-fold higher than her risk of death from breast cancer.[15] Most researchers have concluded that the benefits of HRT on bone and cardiovascular health and generalized feeling of well-being far outweigh the risks.[16,17] Before we have all the answers, you should do monthly self breast exams and have a mammogram before beginning HRT. Once beginning HRT, you should continue with monthly self breast exams and have yearly mammograms and physical exams, ideally staggered at 6-month intervals. The bottom line is that the decision whether or not to use HRT is a very individual one. Each of us must weigh the risks and benefits of such long-term therapy in view of our own personal and family histories of heart disease, cancer, and osteoporosis. Each year we learn more from research, increasing the evidence to sway us more in the direction either for or against HRT use. Regardless of your decision, it is important to reduce all of your other risk factors for osteoporosis, the sooner the better.

Alternatives to HRT

The most widely used non-HRT medications to treat postmenopausal osteoporosis are drugs that either stimulate bone formation or inhibit bone resorption, including the bisphosphonates, calcitonin, vitamin D, fluoride, and thiazide diuretics. These medications act by slowing or reversing the loss of bone mass after menopause, and they may be the ideal alternatives to women who cannot, or choose not to, use HRT.

The *bisphosphonates* act specifically at the sites of bone turnover by binding to the osteoclasts (the cells that break down bone) and inactivating them. *Alendronate,* also known as *Fosamax,* is one of the bisphosphonates. Approved by the Food and Drug Administration in 1995 in a 5-mg dose for the prevention of osteoporosis, this medication slows bone loss and promotes the formation of new bone. The first studies have reported reductions in vertebral and femoral fractures and increases in bone mass in the spine, hip, and total body.[18-20] Alendronate has none of the advantages (or disadvantages) of HRT. Like all medications, alendronate has its drawbacks—it's difficult to digest and hard on the digestive system. It can bind to food and pass through the digestive system unabsorbed; therefore, it must be taken on an empty stomach with plenty of water. Because of these side effects, this medication may not be the best choice for women with swallowing difficulties, heartburn, or ulcers.

Another medication used to treat osteoporosis is *calcitonin.* Available in an injectable form since 1984 and as a nasal spray since 1995, calcitonin is one of the calcium-regulating hormones produced by the thyroid gland. The most common pharmaceutical source of this hormone is from salmon, and the usual daily dose ranges from 50 to 200 IU. Calcitonin has been used to treat women with osteoporosis for about a decade, although its effectiveness is still uncertain.[21-23] Many women who take this medication have a slowing of bone loss and a small increase in bone mass, but it is not as effective as HRT or alendronate in building bone. In addition to such side effects as dizziness, nausea and vomiting, increased urination, and flushing of the face and hands, many individuals may develop a resistance to salmon calcitonin over time. One of the main advantages of this hormone, though, is its ability to relieve bone pain—for this reason, it is often prescribed for women who have already experienced osteoporotic fractures.

As discussed in Chapters One and Two, vitamin D is essential for calcium absorption by the digestive system. As we age, our ability to absorb calcium declines. *Calcitriol* is a more active form of vitamin D, and early results of studies conducted in Europe suggest that this therapy may help reduce the incidence of vertebral fractures in postmenopausal women. Calcitriol is still considered an experimental medication here in the United States, and most researchers agree that more studies need to be conducted, as too much vitamin D can be toxic.

Fluoride is a compound that has been used for decades in drinking water and toothpaste to help prevent tooth decay. Fluoride can stimulate the formation of new bone and increase bone mass, although early experimental trials showed that excessive exposure could cause abnormal bone formation, fractures, and gastric bleeding. More recent studies have used a cyclical, intermittent lower slow-release dose and continuous supplementation with calcium with good results.[24-26] This therapy holds promise for the future.

Thiazide diuretics are medications used primarily to treat high blood pressure and other circulatory conditions. A beneficial side effect of this medication is that it decreases the amount of calcium lost in the urine. Thiazide diuretics help slow bone loss by increasing blood levels of calcium, which in turn signals the parathyroid hormone to reduce the activity of osteoclasts, the specialized cells that break down bone. A growing body of research suggests that thiazide use, particularly in combination with estrogen or HRT, is associated with better bone health among postmenopausal women.[27-34]

On the horizon are several other medications that show promise in research studies in halting or reversing postmenopausal bone changes, but their use has not yet been approved by the Food and Drug Administration. One of these medications is a tissue-specific estrogen, commonly referred to as "designer estrogens." Such a medication would have all the beneficial effects of estrogen on bone, brain, and the cardiovascular system but would not affect uterine or breast tissue. One such medication, *raloxifene,* also known as *Evista,* was approved in 1997 by the Food and Drug Administration in a 60-mg dosage to prevent osteoporosis in postmenopausal women. Originally prescribed to treat breast cancer, raloxifene and a related medication, *tamoxifen,* act by binding to estrogen receptor sites on bone, preventing an immune reaction. The results of current trials will shed light on whether or not these medications might be good alternatives to HRT.

Prescription Medications

For many individuals, acute or chronic health conditions are of a greater immediate concern. Medications prescribed for many of these conditions can have a profound effect on bone health and should be discussed with your physician (see Table 1). The effects of such medications are influenced not only by the state of your bone

TABLE 1
Some Conditions Whose Treatment Can Affect Bone Health
■■

Arthritis	Growth hormone deficiency
Asthma	Heart transplantation
Burn injuries	Hemophilia
Cancer, including leukemia	Hypothyroidism
Cerebral palsy	Inborn errors of metabolism
Crohn's disease	Inflammatory bowel disease
Cystic fibrosis	Muscular dystrophy
Dialysis and renal disease	Thalassemia major
Fractures	Systemic lupus erythematosus

health when the therapy is initiated but also by your age, nutritional status, and the duration of the therapy. Two of the most commonly prescribed medications—corticoid steroids for asthma and thyroid hormone for hypothyroidism—both have an adverse effect on bone health. Although beyond the scope of this book, prescription medications are important to consider when assessing your overall risk for osteoporosis.

Calcium Supplements

As I have discussed earlier, calcium is one of the three key ingredients for building and maintaining good bones throughout our lives. Calcium from food sources has several advantages over calcium from supplements: better bioavailability (more readily absorbed); reduced risk of toxic or teratogenic intakes; presence of other nutrients; improving your overall diet; and reduced cost. But if it is not possible to meet your daily calcium needs through your diet, calcium supplements are a practical alternative. Not all supplements are the same, though. First, avoid buying calcium supplements made from dolomite, bone meal, oyster shells, or other sources labeled as "natural"—these types of supplements are much more likely to contain lead or other toxic metals.[35,36] Second, depending on the form, calcium supplements contain varying amounts of pure, or *elemental,* calcium combined with other substances. For example, the percentage of elemental calcium varies from 40% for calcium carbonate and calcium phosphate, 21% for calcium citrate, 13% for calcium lactate, to 9% for calcium gluconate. Viewed another way, to get 1,000 mg of elemental calcium, you would need to take 2,500 mg of calcium carbonate, 4,750 mg of calcium citrate, 7,700 mg of calcium lactate, or 11,100 mg of calcium gluconate—quite a difference! This translates into having to take more pills to meet your daily calcium requirement.

There are several other considerations when choosing the calcium supplement that's right for you. Absorption is most efficient when at doses of 500 mg or less and when taken with meals. Calcium can interact with other compounds in food, such as iron, and with other medications you might be taking, such as aspirin or tetracycline, interfering with absorption.

Calcium supplements in dosages of less than 2 grams per day do not usually cause side effects, but the most common ones are constipation and gas. When calcium passes through the gastrointestinal system unabsorbed, it causes the stool to become hard. Smaller doses taken with a full glass of water may help, as well as switching to a supplement that also contains magnesium or vitamin D. Gas is frequently caused by the type and form of calcium; calcium carbonate and chewable tablets may be at fault. Also, switching brands may solve the problem. Ask your pharmacist for help in choosing the best calcium supplement for you. My personal favorites are Nature Made Calcium and Magnesium with Zinc and One-A-Day Calcium Plus (with vitamin D and magnesium). The take-home message is that you need adequate calcium every day, and if you are not getting it from your diet, you need to find a supplement that you can stick with in the long run.

In the next chapter we are going to examine the effect of lifestyle choices on bone health—choices we make in our daily lives that may be undermining building good bones. Onward!

CHAPTER 8

The Lifestyle Factors

The Role of Personal Choices in Everyday Life

Bone Basics:

- *One out of four women is a smoker, and 90% of the smokers became regular smokers by age 20.*

- *Women who smoke double their risk of an earlier menopause, by 2–5 years.*

- *Smoking is associated with reduced bone density and increased risk for fractures.*

- *Excessive alcohol use is the number one cause of osteoporosis among men.*

- *Excessive alcohol use in women can result in irregular menstrual cycles, poor nutritional status, and impaired immune response.*

Every day we make choices in our daily lives, from what to wear to what to eat. Many of these choices are part of our daily routine, integrated into our lives as habits—some are healthy, like always buckling up when we get into our cars, and some are unhealthy, like smoking. Still other choices, such as caffeine and alcohol use, can become unhealthy only in excess. In this chapter I'm going to discuss several lifestyle choices that directly affect your bone health: smoking, alcohol, and caffeine. These are all choices completely under your control, and I hope by the time you finish this chapter (and certainly by the time you finish this book!), you will decide to make lifestyle choices with your bone health in mind.

Smoking

If you need another good reason to quit smoking, here it is: it wreaks havoc with your bones! In addition to increasing your risks for heart disease, lung disease, and several types of cancer, smoking also increases your chances of developing osteoporosis. In the United States today, an estimated 48 million adults are smokers, including 25 million men and 23 million women (25% of whom are pregnant).[1,2] Viewed another way, one out of every four women is a smoker, and 90% of the smokers became regular smokers by 20 years of age.[3]

Smoking increases the risk of osteoporosis by at least three mechanisms, maybe more. First, various compounds in cigarette smoke have a toxic effect on the ovaries, causing an irreversible loss of function and accelerated aging. Second, smoking may affect the normal secretion of hormones that regulate the menstrual cycle. Third, smoking alters the metabolism of the sex hormones, primarily estrogen in women and testosterone in men, leading to a decrease in their production and an increase in their conversion to an inactive form.[4]

Smoking also results in nutritional imbalances, which have an indirect adverse effect on bone health. For example, smokers require more than three times the RDA of vitamin C to maintain the same blood levels as nonsmokers.[5] Smokers also have lower levels of vitamins A, B_6, E, and folic acid. Smoking also impairs the activation of vitamin D by the liver, and vitamin D is a crucial player in calcium absorption and bone remodeling.

As a result of these hormonal changes, women who smoke double their risk of an earlier natural menopause, by as much as 2-5 years, compared to women of the same age who never smoked.[6] Because American women can now expect to live more than one-third of their lives after menopause, any risk factor that alters the age at which menopause occurs can have a substantial effect on a woman's health. An analysis of 14 studies of menopause and smoking published between 1966 and 1989 showed that the increased risk of earlier menopause with smoking exists for women as young as 44 years of age; former smokers were found to have a lower risk compared to current smokers, indicating that the effect is at least partially reversible.[6] Even when estrogen is replaced with hormone replacement therapy after menopause, it is not as effective in preventing bone loss among smokers compared to nonsmokers.[7] Consequently, postmenopausal women who smoke require significantly higher doses of hormones.[8]

Cigarette smoking is associated with reduced bone density and increased risk for fractures in later life among both men and women. One study estimated that each decade of smoking is associated with a deficit in spinal bone density of 1.5% and hip bone density of 0.4% to 1.1%.[9] The risk of hip fracture among smokers is double that of nonsmokers.[10] The effect of smoking on bone density is dose-related, with a greater risk of bone loss among heavy smokers, less of a risk among light smokers, and even less of a risk among former smokers.[11] So, if ever there was a time to quit, it's now. Your bones will thank you!

Alcohol

In the United States, about seven out of ten adults consume alcohol, and although men generally drink more frequently and in larger amounts, the proportion of women who drink alcohol has been steadily rising. On a national basis, we drink four times as much alcohol as we do milk. *Among men, alcohol intake is a primary cause of osteoporosis.* Studies have shown a 50% reduction in bone mass among men with chronic alcoholism.[12,13]

Lifestyle factors can reverse positive racial and genetic factors for osteoporosis, even among men. For example, among the Bantu of South Africa, osteoporosis was uncommon, despite lifelong low dietary calcium intakes (averaging 250–400 mg per day), primarily because of a low urinary excretion of calcium.[14,15] Among male Bantu laborers in Johannesburg who developed osteoporosis, heavy drinking, combined with a high iron and low vitamin C intake, were found to be the culprits.[16] Other researchers have also reported an adverse effect of a high alcohol intake on bone health.[17] The alcohol-related hormonal effects in men also include lowered testosterone levels and decreased sperm production.

Women metabolize alcohol differently than men, and this difference has serious health implications. About one-fourth to one-third of alcohol is absorbed in the stomach (gastric absorption); the remainder is absorbed in the small intestine. Gastric absorption is increased by the presence of carbonated fluids and delayed by coldness and the presence of other foods, particularly those high in protein, fat, or sugar. In contrast, the absorption of alcohol in the small intestine occurs very rapidly, regardless of the presence of food. Men and women differ in their ability to absorb alcohol, with women having less gastric absorption and more rapid and complete absorption in the small intestine.[18] Because of this difference, women are more susceptible to the effects of alcohol, more likely to have a higher blood alcohol content (become drunk quicker) from the same amount, and suffer more long-term physical damage from its effects.[19-22] Alcohol alters the body's normal hormonal balance, and the results have widespread consequences for nearly every system in the body, including the bones.[23] Women who drink two or more drinks per day can suffer significant disturbances in their menstrual cycles and even infertility, decreased ability to breast-feed, muscle weakness, altered carbohydrate metabolism, damage to heart tissue, and impaired immune response.

Alcohol affects bone health in direct and indirect ways. Alcohol is believed to act directly by inhibiting the function of the bone-forming cells, the osteoblasts.[24,25] Indirectly, alcohol impairs vitamin D metabolism and the absorption of calcium from the upper part of the gastrointestinal tract. As will be discussed in Chapter 9, "The Nutrient Factors," vitamin D is formed primarily in the skin in the presence of sunlight; smaller amounts are also obtained through the diet in the form of enriched dairy products. Vitamin D is first metabolized to a more active form by the liver and then to its most potent form by the kidneys, under the control of parathyroid hormone. This most active form of vitamin D (officially termed *1,25-dihydroxycholecalciferol* or *calcitriol*) is responsible for the regulation of calcium absorption from the gastrointestinal tract. Alcohol impairs this absorption, leading to a fall in serum calcium levels and the demineralization of calcium from the bones. As recommended in the most recent *Dietary Guidelines for Americans,*[26] if you drink alcoholic beverages, do so in moderation, which translates as no more than one drink per day for women and no more than two drinks per day for men.

Caffeine

The scientific evidence is strong between smoking, drinking, and poor bone health, but the jury is still out when it comes to caffeine. Some studies have reported caffeine intake to be a risk factor,[27-30] while others have not.[31-33] Let's look at the facts. Caffeine is a naturally occurring substance found in the leaves, seeds, or fruit of many types of plants, including coffee beans, cocoa beans, cola nuts, and tea leaves. We enjoy many foods that contain varying amounts of caffeine, but for most of us the most common and concentrated source is coffee.

Caffeine's connection with bone health is through calcium, via the kidneys. Every day we lose a cetain amount of calcium via our kidneys (termed **obligatory losses**). Certain factors can increase those losses, including high intakes of sodium (from table salt and processed foods) and phosphates (from sodas and proteins); we will look at these factors more closely in Chapter 9, "The Nutrient Factors." But caffeine has been implicated as another factor in our daily diets that can also increase urinary losses of calcium, potentially pulling this vital mineral from our bones. Several studies have reported that caffeine increases urinary losses of calcium, but this effect occurred only during the first few hours after intake.[29] In addition, this increased urinary loss of calcium was more likely to occur among women with low calcium intakes.

The most recent and most carefully conducted studies to date do not show any significant effect of caffeine on bone health.[31-33] One study analyzed caffeine intake by both diet records and gas chromatography of each subject's brewed caffeinated beverages, and found no link between habitual dietary caffeine intake and bone health.[32] Another study concluded that caffeine intakes of 400 mg or less do not increase urinary losses of calcium, provided the dietary intake of calcium was at least 600 mg.[31] Current scientific evidence suggests that moderate caffeine intake does not increase a woman's risk for developing osteoporosis, at least if her calcium intake is adequate. So, the bottom line is, limit your daily intake of caffeine (or switch to decaffeinated) and make sure you get enough calcium every day. In Table 1, I've listed some common sources of caffeine.

The message regarding good bones and lifestyle is, "Quit smoking, and if you choose to drink alcohol or caffeinated beverages, do so in moderation." In the next two chapters I'm going to give you a crash course in foods and nutrition: the very foundation of life, and certainly the cornerstone of good bone health. Let's begin.

Food	Amount	Caffeine (mg)
Brewed coffee	6 fl. oz.	90–100
Ground coffee	1 tbsp.	
Chocolate chips	6 oz.	
Coca-Cola, regular or diet	12 fl. oz.	40–60
Cherry Coke, regular or diet	12 fl. oz.	
Dr. Pepper, regular or diet	12 fl. oz.	
Diet-Rite Cola	12 fl. oz.	
Mello Yello	12 fl. oz.	
Powdered instant coffee	1 rounded tsp.	
Pepsi-Cola, regular or diet	12 fl. oz.	30–40
Brewed tea	6 fl. oz.	
Instant tea	1 tsp.	
Hershey's Special Dark Chocolate	1.45-oz. bar	
RC Cola, regular or cherry	12 fl. oz.	10–20
Semisweet chocolate	1 oz.	
Chocolate chips	1/4 cup	
Nestlé Crunch bar	1.4-oz. bar	
Mars Milky Way bar	2.1-oz. bar	
Hershey's KitKat bar	1.6-oz. bar	<10
Reese's Peanut Butter Cups	1.8-oz bar	
Brownies	1 oz.	
Devil's food cake	1/12 cake	
Chocolate pudding	1/2 cup	
Chocolate chip cookies	2 medium	

CHAPTER 9

The Nutrient Factors

Translating Research into Reality

Bone Basics:

- *One out of two American children gets less than 400 mg of dietary calcium per day.*
- *From childhood to adolescence, the dietary calcium requirement doubles.*
- *Three out of four American women get less than 800 mg of dietary calcium per day.*
- *At menopause, calcium requirements increase by 500 mg per day.*
- *Protein and sodium in the diet can dramatically influence calcium requirements.*
- *Dietary fiber increases the calcium requirement by 100 mg per 18 mg of fiber.*
- *Calcium reduces the availability and absorption of both iron and zinc.*

Calcium is at the very heart of the issue of healthy bones, but how much is enough? And how much is too much? What are the best sources, and do we all need the same amount? These and many other important questions have been addressed by research scientists around the world, and we now have answers. Because the issue of nutrition is so important, and because it involves both the science of how our bodies utilize nutrients and the art of choosing the right foods to meet our needs, I have divided up this information into two chapters. In this chapter we will first address the nutrient factors, the science of nutrition; identify factors influencing how much calcium we need; and determine our calcium requirement. In the next chapter I will address how to put this knowledge to work when making food choices at home and at work, when eating out or dining in, including how to use food labeling to get the best nutrition. Let's begin.

What Are Americans Eating?

Since our bodies can not make calcium, the main ingredient in bones, we must get it from our diets. But are we getting enough calcium for healthy bones? Not the average American. Today we drink about three-fourths the amount of milk, the primary source of dietary calcium, as we did in 1970—averaging little more than a glass a day, or about a quart a week. In contrast, on a national basis we drink about three quarts a week of beer, wine, and distilled spirits and about four quarts a week of soft drinks.[1] Current national surveys indicate that not only are women not drinking enough milk, but they generally have diets that are severely inadequate in many nutrients, including calcium. The majority of American women have diets containing less than 67% of the RDA for calcium, including three out of four women aged 19-24 and one out of two women aged 25 and older.[2] In addition, more than half of American children have diets that provide less than 50% of the RDAs for calcium, setting the stage for lower peak bone mass by adulthood and increasing their likelihood of developing osteoporosis when they reach their forties, fifties and beyond.[3]

The skeleton is more than just calcium—a balance of many elements is needed to build and maintain strong, healthy bones. In addition, your calcium requirement depends on your other risk factors, including other dietary factors. The single most important nondietary factor affecting calcium absorption is your age. During periods of rapid growth, such as infancy, adolescence, and pregnancy, the absorption of calcium may be quite high. But after adolescence, that absorption drops to about 20-40% among young adults, and it declines even further as we age. When the level of calcium in the diet is low, a higher percentage is absorbed. Dietary factors affect your calcium requirement by influencing either absorption by the gastrointestinal tract or excretion by the kidneys. Let's review how the other aspects of your daily diet influence your optimal level of calcium.

Factors Influencing Calcium Absorption

The factors influencing the absorption of calcium by the gastrointestinal tract include vitamin D, dietary fiber, binding agents, lactose and dairy products, and certain diseases and types of surgery.

Vitamin D

Vitamin D is important for bone health because of its role in promoting calcium absorption and its positive interaction with other bone-building hormones. Vitamin D is formed in the skin when its precursor absorbs ultraviolet light from sunshine. As discussed in Chapter 3, "The Heredity Factors," the amount of vitamin D produced on exposure to sunshine depends on skin pigment, as well as length of exposure. Darker-skinned people require a longer period of exposure, because less ultraviolet light is able to penetrate. It's not possible to overdose on this vitamin from exposure to sunshine, because we have a built-in mechanism that turns off vitamin D production when 15-20% of the precursor stores have been converted to the active form. But overdosing is a real possibility when it comes to supplements of this vitamin. To prevent vitamin D deficiency, all milk sold in the United States is fortified at the level of 400 IU per quart; other dairy products do not contain this fortification. In other countries, margarine is fortified with vitamin D. Other sources of this essential bone-building vitamin include salmon, tuna, shrimp, liver, and egg yolk.

Dietary fiber

Dietary fiber is a type of carbohydrate, found in certain foods, that is not absorbed by the body and passes undigested through the gastrointestinal tract. Changes in food labeling have made it easier to identify sources of dietary fiber (see Chapter 10), which has received increasing importance as a healthy part of our daily diet. For example, one of the national health objectives for the year 2000 is to increase fiber-containing foods in the adult diet to five or more servings per day, and the most recent revision of **Dietary Guidelines for Americans** (graphically presented as the **Food Guide Pyramid**) recommends 2-4 servings per day of fruits and 3-5 servings per day of vegetables, both rich sources of dietary fiber.[4,5] Recent national surveys indicate that only one out of three Americans is meeting the five-a-day guidelines, only one out of four meets the guidelines for fruits, and one out of eight for vegetables.[6]

Other surveys have reported that Americans are eating less than half the recommended 6–11 servings per day of grain foods (breads, cereal, rice, and pasta), another rich source of dietary fiber.[7] The dietary fiber content of common foods is given in Table 1.

Mounting scientific evidence has linked the presence of these indigestible carbohydrates with reductions in heart disease, cancer, and diabetes. Dietary fiber may lower the risk of heart disease by decreasing the time it takes for food to travel through the gastrointestinal tract, reducing the absorption of dietary fat and cholesterol and thereby lowering serum cholesterol levels. Fiber's protective role against colon cancer is also linked to its ability to move digested food more rapidly through the large intestine, reducing exposure to potential cancer-causing substances. In addition, by absorbing fluids as they are digested, dietary fiber may also act by diluting the concentration of these toxic substances. The exact mechanism of how dietary fiber improves blood sugar levels among diabetics is still unclear, but it seems to play a positive role. The negative aspect of dietary fiber is its ability to bind minerals, specifically calcium, and prevent their absorption. The dietary fiber in grains and grain products (cereals, breads) does reduce calcium absorption, whereas the dietary fiber in fruits and vegetables has no effect. It is recommended that the calcium requirement be increased by 100 mg for each 18 grams of dietary fiber.

Binding agents

Several dietary factors, including *oxalates, phytates, phosphates,* and *fats,* bind calcium to some degree, preventing it from being absorbed. Oxalates are found in spinach, rhubarb, and cocoa; phytates are present in cereal grains; and phosphates are present in processed foods and soft drinks. Although food labels list the calcium content of a particular food, that amount has been determined in a laboratory and is not the most accurate estimate of how much is available for absorption or is eventually absorbed by the body. For example, compared to the calcium in milk, the calcium in kidney beans is only about half as available, while the calcium in spinach and rhubarb is nearly completely unavailable. Keep this in mind

TABLE 1

Food		Amount	Dietary Fiber (grams)
Breads and Cereals	Fiber One, General Mills	1 oz (1/2 c)	13.0
	All-Bran, Kellogg's	1 oz (1/2 c)	10.0
	Bran Buds, Kellogg's	1 oz (1/2 c)	8.0
	Bran Chex, Ralston Purina	1 oz (2/3 c)	6.1
	Cracklin Oat Bran, Kellogg's	1 oz (1/3 c)	4.0
	Grape-Nuts, Post	1 oz (1/4 c)	2.6
	Cheerios, General Mills	1 oz (1 1/4 c)	2.0
	Whole Wheat Bread	1 slice	1.6
	Cracked Wheat Bread	1 slice	1.1
	White Bread	1 slice	0.8
	Oatmeal Bread	1 slice	0.6
	Raisin Bread	1 slice	0.6
Fruits and Vegetables	Pear	1 medium	4.3
	Strawberries	1 cup	3.9
	Pumpkin, canned	1/2 c	3.8
	Apples	1 medium	3.0
	Oranges	1 medium	2.9

TABLE 1 (continued)

Food	Amount	Dietary Fiber (grams)
Fruits and Vegetables (cont.)		
Squash, baked	1/2 c	2.9
Peas, cooked	1/2 c	2.2
Broccoli, cooked	1/2 c	2.0
Bananas	1 medium	1.8
Cabbage, cooked	1/2 c	1.8
Carrots, cooked	1/2 c	1.5
Cauliflower, cooked	1/2 c	1.4
Peaches	1 medium	1.4
Onions, raw	1/2 c	1.2
Corn, canned	1/2 c	1.1
Cherries, fresh	10	1.1
Nuts and Legumes		
Three bean salad	1/2 c	3.2
Almonds, dry roasted	1 oz	3.1
Chickpeas	1/2 c	2.9
Peanuts, dry roasted	1 oz	2.2
Cashews	1 oz	1.7
Green beans, cooked	1/2 c	1.1

when choosing dietary sources of calcium, and limit foods with calcium-binding factors.

Fat, the most concentrated source of energy in our diets, can also bind calcium and prevent its absorption. National health and nutrition guidelines recommend limiting fat intake to 30% or less of total calories (67 grams/day with 2,000 calories; 60 grams/day with 1,800 calories). Recent dietary surveys suggest that Americans are reducing their fat intakes, although this is not a universal finding among all age groups.[8-11]

Lactose and dairy products

Lactose, the double-ringed carbohydrate found exclusively in milk and milk products, is an important player in the calcium story. This unique carbohydrate enhances absorption by binding to calcium and preventing other elements in the diet from interfering with its absorption. Because lactose is slowly broken down during digestion, it helps acidify the environment in the small intestine, further aiding calcium absorption. Milk and milk products provide about 75% of the calcium in our diets.

Although milk and milk products are traditionally considered the primary sources of dietary calcium, the majority of the world's adult population is unable to digest varying quantities of milk because of a low level of the enzyme *lactase.* This enzyme, located in the small intestines, is responsible for the breakdown of lactose to the single-ringed sugars glucose and galactose. Only single-ringed sugars can be absorbed, so if the capacity of the available lactase is exceeded (when more lactose is ingested than can be broken down), the undigested lactose passes into the large intestine, the colon. This undigested lactose is fermented by bacteria present in the colon; in addition to pulling in fluids from the surrounding tissues, this fermentation causes the classic symptoms of lactose intolerance: abdominal cramps, bloating, diarrhea, and gas.

There are several strategies for coping with lactose intolerance while still getting the calcium you need. First, determine how much lactose produces symptoms for you. Second, eat dairy products with a snack or meal, slowing down digestion and therefore reducing symptoms; several studies have shown that this method alleviates symptoms.[12-15] Third, include dairy products in which the lactose has been reduced during processing, such as aged hard cheeses or specially formulated lactose-reduced or lactose-free milks. This second choice often is available in a calcium-fortified form, providing 500 mg of calcium in a single 8-ounce serving. Yogurt is also a good choice, but for a different reason. The active cultures in many types of yogurt provide an alternative enzyme source to break down lactose; look for the phrase "active cultures present" on the label. A fourth alternative is to add an enzyme directly to milk to reduce or eliminate the lactose that is present. These enzyme preparations are available in local pharmacies and grocery stores and are simple to use. Treated milk, as well as the specially formulated milks, taste sweeter than regular milk because the lactose is broken down into sweeter-tasting single-ringed carbohydrates. These enzyme preparations are also available in tablet form, releasing the lactase enzyme in your stomach so that it can work while you eat.

Dairy products and bone health

Several studies have specifically examined the relationship between the consumption of dairy products and current and long-term bone health. These studies have shown that calcium intake through milk and milk products during childhood and adolescence improves bone mass and bone density during adolescence,[16] during young adulthood (ages 25–30),[17] and after menopause.[18,19] Differences in calcium nutrition during childhood and adolescence are estimated to account for as much as 5–10% difference in peak bone mass, which in turn contributes to more than 50% of the difference in hip fracture rates later in life.[20-23] The unique combination of nutrients in milk may be particularly beneficial for bone development, and, as these studies show, including dairy products as a regular part of your diet is a wise investment in your bone health.

Diseases and surgery

Any disease or surgery that disrupts the integrity of the small intestine, the main site of calcium absorption, will result in decreased absorption and increased losses of dietary calcium. Examples include such conditions as malabsorption syndromes, primary biliary cirrhosis, and celiac disease. Individuals who have undergone a partial gastrectomy frequently have decreased calcium absorption due to malabsorption of vitamin D. Individuals who have had intestinal resection for obesity also have malabsorption of both calcium and vitamin D, but the body accommodates through growth of the remaining gut. Any surgery on the gastrointestinal tract can potentially alter calcium absorption and should be considered in the overall management.

Factors Influencing Calcium Excretion

The primary factors influencing the urinary loss of calcium include the dietary levels of protein and sodium. Together, they outweigh all the other dietary factors that influence absorption. Getting the right amount of protein in your diet is also an important part of building and maintaining good bones: the skeleton is second only to muscle in terms of total protein content. It may surprise you to learn that too much protein in your diet, as well as too little, can result in a loss of bone mass. When your diet is too high in protein, the kidneys excrete more calcium, pulling calcium already laid down in the bones. A high level of protein is about twice the RDA, or about 100 grams or more for adult women and 150 grams or more for adult men. Every gram of protein metabolized by the body causes the urinary loss of 1 mg of calcium.

Dietary sodium

If your diet is too high in sodium, it can result in increased urinary losses of calcium. The average daily sodium intake for American children ages three and older is 2,400 mg, and for women is about 3,000 mg; our minimum needs are only about 500 mg. Every 2,000 mg of sodium excreted by the kidneys pulls 10-30 mg of calcium out with it. Habitually high intakes of sodium may be a significant factor in the development of kidney stones. Researchers have found that individuals who are prone to developing kidney stones excrete twice as much calcium at the same sodium intake as those who do not develop kidney stones.[24] At low sodium and protein intakes, the calcium requirement to maintain balance for the average woman may be as little as 400 mg per day, but if her intake of both sodium and protein is high, she might require as much as 2,000 mg of calcium per day. This effect of sodium and protein on calcium balance, and therefore calcium requirements, in large part explains differences between populations around the world. In the United States, our generally high intakes of both of sodium and protein increase our optimal level of calcium in our diets, which is typically low.

Interaction with Other Nutrients

Calcium itself can reduce the absorption of other nutrients in the diet, including iron and zinc. When included at the same meal, calcium reduces the availability and absorption of both iron and zinc, increasing their requirements.[25-27] When calcium-rich foods or calcium supplements are taken separately from iron or zinc, absorption of all three minerals is improved.[28]

The Calcium Requirement

With all of these factors in mind, it's time to look at the calcium requirement—how much we need at every age. As discussed earlier, calcium absorption decreases with age. From birth to about age 10, bone mass increases from about 25 grams to 390-450 grams. After infancy, the absorption of dietary calcium averages 35-45%, putting the amount of dietary calcium necessary to support this linear increase at about 550-650 mg per day. Allowing for a mixed diet and individual variation, the estimated daily requirement for calcium is about 800-1,200 mg.

During adolescence, skeletal growth accelerates, doubling the calcium requirements of childhood. Although calcium absorption increases to about 40-45% during this period, urinary losses increase with age, setting the daily calcium requirement to 1,400-1,600 mg.[29,30] This level is supported by recent studies demonstrating that urinary losses of calcium did not increase significantly, even with dietary intakes of calcium as high as 1,600 mg per day.[31] Even at this level of dietary calcium, the capacity of the growing skeleton has not been reached: calcium retention by the skeleton continues to increase at dietary intakes over 2,000 mg per day.[30] Because the average daily retention rate during adolescence is at least twice that during childhood, it has been recommended by scientists and researchers that the calcium requirement also be at least twice the childhood level (see Table 2).

During the twenties and thirties, skeletal growth continues, but at a slower rate. Calcium absorption is about 30-35% in this age group, and a daily calcium intake of about 1,200 mg should be adequate. Between age 30 and menopause, a woman's calcium requirement is about 1,000 mg per day. Maintaining an adequate daily intake of calcium is still important during this stage of life, even though growth is completed and the mechanisms for conserving acquired bone mass are still relatively efficient. Daily calcium intakes above this level (1,000 mg per day) have been shown to be therapeutic in preventing bone loss. In one study, premenopausal women with average dietary intakes of 900 mg of calcium per day were shown to be losing bone from the lumbar spine at the rate of nearly 1% per year, compared to no bone loss among a second group who were additionally supplemented with 600 mg of calcium per day.[32]

During the time around menopause, there is a rapid loss of bone mass, with the sudden drop in the bone-sparing hormone estrogen. This loss occurs within a 3-5 year period, after which calcium balance stabilizes. Estrogen deficiency further reduces calcium absorption and, combined with the increasing urinary losses due to aging, results in a calcium requirement for the woman not receiving hormone replacement therapy of about 1,500-1,700 mg per day.

The estrogen deprivation effect appears to increase the calcium requirement by about 500 mg per day. Therefore, for adults aged 25-65 the calcium requirement is 1,000-1,200 mg per day for men, premenopausal women, and postmenopausal women in conjunction with hormone replacement therapy, and 1,500-1,700 mg per day for postmenopausal women in the absence of estrogen replacement.[33] For men and women aged 65 and older, the calcium requirement is 1,500 mg per day.

Table 2 summarizes recommendations from the Food and Nutrition Board of the National Research Council (the RDAs),[34] the National Institutes of Health (NIH) Consensus Development Conference (1994), recent revisions from the Institute of Medicine (IOM),[35] and major researchers and scientists involved in studies of bone health.

Although the jury is still out regarding the precise amount of calcium we need every day, one thing is clear from looking at Table 2: we all need calcium, and probably more than what we are getting. Adolescence is the most critical period, with many experts suggesting daily intakes of over 1,500 mg. Young adults need close to this amount, as well as women who are pregnant or breast-feeding. Our requirements rise again around menopause and stay at this level for the rest of our lives. Now that we've determined how much calcium we need, where do we get it? In the next chapter we will apply what we've learned here, to make the best food choices for healthy bones. Let's begin.

TABLE 2
Summary of Daily Calcium Requirements (mg)

Age Group	RDAs, 1989	NIH, 1994	IOM, 1998	Johnston et al, 1992 ref. 36	Jackman et al, 1997 ref. 30	Matkovic & Heaney, 1992 ref. 31	Chapuy et al, 1992, ref. 38 Heaney et al, 1989, ref. 39
Infants							
Birth–6 months	400	400	210				
6 months–1 year	600	600	270				
Children							
1	800	800	500			1,100	
2–3	800	800	500			1,100	
4–5	800	800	800			1,100	
6	800	800–1,200	800			1,100	
7–8	800	800–1,200	800	1,600		1,100	
Adolescents							
9–10	800	800–1,200	1,300	1,600		1,600	
11–12	1,200	1,200–1,500	1,300	1,600	1,300–2,100	1,600	
13	1,200	1,200–1,500	1,300	1,600	1,300–2,100	1,600	
14	1,200	1,200–1,500	1,300	1,600	1,300–2,100	1,600	
15–18	1,200	1,200–1,500	1,300	1,600		1,600	

TABLE 2 (continued)

Adult women

19–24	1,200	1,200–1,500	1,000	1,100	
25–30	800	1,000	1,000	1,100	
31–50	800	1,000	1,000		
51–65	800		1,200		
On estrogen		1,000			
Not on estrogens		1,500			1,500–1,700
65–70	800	1,500	1,200		
70+	800	1,500	1,200		
Pregnant	1,200	1,200–1,500	1,000		
Lactating	1,200	1,200–1,500	1,000		

Men

19–24	1,200	1,200–1,500	1,000		
25–30	800	1,000	1,000		
31–50	800	1,000	1,000		
51–65	800	1,000	1,200		
65–70	800	1,500	1,200		
70+	800	1,500	1,200		

CHAPTER 10

The Food Factors

The Best Choices for Good Health

Bone Basics:

- *Per capita consumption of milk in the United States is about one glass per day.*

- *As a nation, we drink nearly twice as much beer and wine as we do milk.*

- *With the newest food labeling, Percent Daily Value replaces the U.S. RDA.*

- *For a food manufacturer to make a calcium-osteoporosis health claim, the product must contain at least 200 mg of calcium per serving.*

When Mary, age 48, was growing up, a typical dinner included meat and potatoes, a salad, bread and butter, milk, and layer cake for dessert. Today, when she sits down to dinner with her own family, she's more likely to serve beef stir-fry or have ordered out for pizza; beverages might include sodas for the kids and mineral water or wine for her and her husband. Dessert might be the newest ice cream or cannolis from the Italian pastry shop down the street. Our tastes have changed as a nation, too, with a wider variety of foods now a regular part of our daily lives. We have generally become more health-conscious, although there is still a considerable gap between what we know is good for us and what we choose to eat. Let's take a closer look at how the American diet has changed over the past 25 years, and how we can make it more "bone-healthy."

How We've Changed Our Food Thinking

Thanks primarily to the widespread and persistent efforts of the American Heart Association over the past three decades, as Americans we have become more health-conscious about the foods we eat, and more foods than ever are nutritionally labeled, particularly for fat, saturated fat, cholesterol, and sodium. According to the annual consumer attitude survey conducted by the Food Marketing Institute in Washington, DC, more than seven out of ten consumers consider nutrition very important when buying groceries, out-weighing product safety and even price. More than nine out of ten shoppers have changed their eating habits to try to make their diets more healthful, by including more fruits, vegetables, and poultry and less fats and oils, red meats, snack foods, sugar, butter, cheese, and whole milk.

How We've Changed Our Food Choices

These attitude changes reported by consumers are reflected by behavioral changes. For example, during the past twenty-five years Americans have cut down on three major sources of fat and cho-lesterol in their diets: eggs, butter, and red meat. In addition, Americans have begun to eat more lower-fat, lower-cholesterol foods such as seafood and poultry. Although we are eating more fresh fruits and vegetables, we are also using more salad oil and cooking oil and eating more high-fat dairy products, such as cream, sour cream, and ice cream. In addition, although the aver-age American is drinking less distilled spirits, we are drinking more wine (about seven ounces per week) and beer (about two-thirds of a gallon per week). Obviously, not all food choices are based on nutrition. According to the Food Marketing Institute's annual consumer survey, taste is the single most important con-sideration in buying food, ranked number one by nine out of ten survey respondents.

Calcium-Rich Foods and Health

American consumers appear to have gotten the message regarding fat, cholesterol, and heart disease but are not making the connec-tion between dietary calcium and bone health. The consumption of milk, traditionally the major source of calcium in the American diet, has fallen dramatically over the past 25 years. Sales of whole milk have fallen by two-thirds during this time period, while those of skim milk have doubled and those of low-fat milk tripled, yet when all the numbers are totaled, the average American today only drinks about a glass of milk a day. And although sales of such low-fat, high-calcium foods as yogurt have increased fourfold over this same period, the average American is eating only about one serving per week. Milk and milk products account for more than 75% of the calcium in the U.S. food supply, but they contribute only about half that amount to the diets of adult women. Recent national dietary surveys show that adult women average 600 mg or less of calcium per day, or about 60% of their actual needs, and only 40% of that calcium is from milk and milk products.[1,2] In addition, more than half of American children and adolescents have diets that provide less than 50% of the RDA for calcium, setting the stage for lower peak bone mass by adulthood and increasing their likelihood of developing osteoporosis when they reach their forties or fifties and beyond.[3]

This national avoidance of dairy products, because of their traditionally high fat and cholesterol content, is no longer necessary.

TABLE 1

■■

Nutrient	Mandatory	Voluntary
Calories	Total calories	
	Calories from fat	Calories from saturated fat
Fat	Total fat	Polyunsaturated fat
	Saturated fat	Monounsaturated fat
Cholesterol	Cholesterol	
Sodium	Sodium	Potassium
Carbohydrate	Total carbohydrate	Soluble fiber
	Dietary fiber	Insoluble fiber
	Sugars	Sugar alcohols
Protein	Protein	
Vitamins	Vitamin A	
	Vitamin C	
Minerals	Calcium	
	Iron	

FIGURE 1
Example of the new food label
▪▪▪▪▪▪▪▪▪▪▪▪▪▪▪▪▪▪▪▪▪▪▪▪▪▪▪▪▪▪▪▪▪▪▪▪

Nutrition Facts	Amount/Serving	%DV*	Amount/Serving	%DV*
Serv. Size 1 oz (28g) Servings Varied Calories 100 Fat Cal. 70	Total Fat 8g	12%	Total Carb. 0g	0%
	Sat. Fat 5g	25%	Fiber 0g	0%
	Cholest 30mg	10%	Sugars 0g	
*Percent Daily Values (DV) are based on a 2,000 calorie diet.	Sodium 180mg	8%	Protein 7g	
	Vitamin A 6% • Vitamin C 0% • Calcium 20% • Iron 0%			

There are more choices in the dairy case than ever before that are both "bone-healthy" and "heart-healthy." Dairy products are still the best sources of calcium, and in today's dairy case it's easier than ever to meet your calcium needs. The array of choices and the terminology can be a bit confusing and even overwhelming at times. So first, let's brush up on how to decipher food labels—the key to making the best food choices.

Food Labeling: The Key to Good Nutrition

In 1993, the Food and Drug Administration (the FDA) and the U.S. Department of Agriculture's Food Safety and Inspection Service (the FSIS) published revised regulations on food labeling.[4] These regulations, which are a revision of the Nutrition Labeling and Education Act of 1990, call for mandatory labeling of processed foods, meat, and poultry products, and the voluntary provision of nutrition information for fresh fruits and vegetables, and for raw fish at point of purchase. An example of the new labeling format is shown in Figure 1. The mandatory and voluntary components and the order in which they must appear on the FDA-regulated foods are shown in Table 1.

Each of the mandatory nutrients is listed on the label in amounts per serving, as well as in *Percent of Daily Value,* which replaces the term *U.S. RDA* as a reference value. For calcium, the Daily Value is 1,000 mg, so if a serving of a particular food provides

20% of the daily value for calcium, it contains 200 mg. Also included in the new labeling are *Daily Reference Values,* based on an ideal, nutritionally balanced diet supplying either 2,000 or 2,500 calories, with

- Fat based on 30% of calories, with an upper limit of less than 65 grams
- Saturated fat based on 10% of calories, with an upper limit of less than 20 grams
- Cholesterol of less than 300 mg
- Carbohydrate based on 60% of calories
- Protein based on 10% of calories
- Fiber based on 11.5 grams per 1,000 calories
- Sodium less than 2,400 mg

The New Labeling Vocabulary

Several new terms have been introduced with this labeling revision, including *free, low, lean* and *extra lean, high, good source, reduced, less,* and *light* or *lite,* in addition to seven health claims. The term *free* means that a food product contains no, or a trivial amount, of one or more of the following components: fat, saturated fat, cholesterol, sodium, or calories. Synonyms for *free* include *without, no,* and *zero.* The term *low* is permitted in food labeling if a food contains, per serving, 3 grams or less of fat ("low fat"); 1 gram or less of saturated fat ("low saturated fat"); 140 mg or less of sodium ("low sodium"); 35 mg or less of sodium ("very low sodium"); less than 20 mg of cholesterol ("low cholesterol"); or 40 calories or less ("low calorie"). Synonyms for *low* include *low source of, little,* and *few.*

The terms *lean* and *extra lean* may be used to describe the fat content of meat, poultry, seafood, and game meats. *Lean* can be used when, per serving, the food contains less than 10 grams of fat, less than 4 grams of saturated fat, and less than 95 mg of cholesterol. *Extra lean* can be used when, per serving, the food contains less than 5 grams of fat, less than 2 grams of saturated fat, and less than 95 mg of cholesterol.

The term *high* may be used if a food contains 20% or more of the Daily Value for a particular nutrient in a serving. *Good source* indicates that one serving of a food contains 10–19% of the Daily Value for a particular nutrient.

Reduced or *fewer* may be used when a nutritionally altered food contains 25% less of a nutrient or calories than the regular product. The term *less* can be used when a food contains 25% less of a nutrient or calories compared to a reference food. An example of this would be that pretzels contain 25% less fat than potato chips. The term *light* (or *lite*) can be used in two contexts: first, that a nutritionally altered food contains one-third fewer calories or half the fat of the reference food, and second, that the sodium content of a low-calorie, low-fat food has been reduced by 50%.

To make milk labels more in line with other food products, and in response to the milk industry and requests from consumer groups to make it easier to identify low-fat and fat-free milk, the FDA has issued more recent regulations. These specify that, by January 1998, skim or nonfat milk will be labeled *fat free;* 1% lowfat milk will be labeled either *low fat* or *light;* 2% lowfat milk will be labeled *reduced fat milk;* whole milk will still be labeled as whole milk.

Truth in Advertising

For the first time, the FDA will allow manufacturers to make certain health claims linking the effect of a nutrient or a food and the risk of a disease or health-related condition. They can be made through third-party references, such as the National Cancer Institute or the American Heart Association; through symbols, such as a heart; and through descriptions. The following is a list of the nutrient-disease relationship claims that are now allowed on food labels:

- Adequate calcium and lowered risk of osteoporosis
- Lowered fat and lowered risk of cancer
- Lowered saturated fat, cholesterol, and lowered risk of coronary heart disease

- Higher fiber-containing fruits, vegetables, and grain products and lowered risk of cancer
- Higher fiber-containing fruits, vegetables, and grain products and lowered risk of coronary heart disease
- Lower sodium and lowered risk of hypertension
- Higher fruits and vegetables and lower risk of cancer
- Adequate intake of folic acid–rich foods before and during pregnancy and a lowered risk of neural tube birth defects

In order for a food product to include the authorized calcium-osteoporosis health claim, the regulations specify that the food (1) be a "high" source of calcium: it must contain, per serving, at least 200 mg of calcium (20% of the daily value); (2) contain a form of calcium that can be readily digested and utilized by the body; and (3) not contain excessive amounts of phosphorus.[5] In other words, you should have confidence that when you buy a food labeled "high calcium," or with the calcium-osteoporosis health claim, that there is truth in advertising, and you are getting good nutrition.

Shopping for Good Nutrition

How can you meet your calcium needs? As I said earlier, the richest sources of calcium are found in dairy products, and with all the innovations in the dairy industry, it's easier than ever to find foods that are "bone-healthy" and heart-healthy." I've done some comparison food shopping to get you started and to apply the new food labeling vocabulary. Remember, these food lists are just examples of the range of food products you can find in your local store, and every day new products are introduced. The choices should not be overwhelming if you are armed with the basic nutrition and labeling knowledge. Studies have shown that the new labeling makes it much easier for consumers to choose nutritious foods.[6] Let's begin with milk (Table 2).

Basically, there are four types of traditional milk, and many more varieties that are either calcium-fortified, lactose-reduced, or rice- or soy-based. Lactose, a type of carbohydrate found only in

TABLE 2
Milk and Milk Products

▪ ▪

Product	Amount	Calories	Fat (g)	Protein (g)	Calcium (mg)
Cow's Milk					
Whole Milk	8 oz.	150	8	8	300
Canned evaporated (reconstituted)	8 oz.	170	9.5	8	330
Reduced Fat Milk	8 oz.	120	5	8	300
Dairy Ease 100 2% fat	8 oz.	130	5	8	300
Lactaid 100 2% fat	8 oz.	130	5	8	300
Lowfat Milk (1%)	8 oz.	100	2.5	8	300
Canned evaporated lowfat (reconstituted)	8 oz.	110	3	9	320
Dairy Ease 100 1% fat	8 oz.	110	2.5	8	300
Lactaid 100 1% fat	8 oz.	110	2.5	8	300
Fat-Free Milk (skim, nonfat)	8 oz.	80	0	8	300
Dry nonfat, reconstituted	8 oz.	80	0	8	300
Dairy Ease 100 nonfat	8 oz.	90	0.5	8	300
Lactaid 100 nonfat	8 oz.	90	0	9	300
Lactaid 100 nonfat, calcium-fortified	8 oz.	80	0	8	500
Fat-Free Milk with Additives					
Ovaltine with 8 oz. fat free milk	8 oz.	160	0	8	380
Alba Dairy Shake Mix with 8 oz. fat-free milk	8 oz.	150	0	14	600
Carnation Instant Breakfast with 8 oz. skim milk	8 oz.	210	1	12	600
Rice and Soy Milks					
White Wave Silk (soy) 1% fat	8 oz.	80	2.5	4	300
White Wave Rice Silk 1% fat	8 oz.	90	2.5	2	300
Eden Soy, Original	8 oz.	130	4	10	80
Eden Soy, Extra	8 oz.	150	3	6	200
Eden Blend Rice and Soy	8 oz.	120	3	7	40
Rice Dream, Organic Original	8 oz.	120	2	1	20
Rice Dream, Organic Original, Enriched	8 oz.	120	2	1	300

dairy products, is difficult for many adults to digest, as discussed in the previous chapter. Lactaid 100® and Dairy Ease 100® are two types of fresh milks in which the lactose has been broken down— these milks are a little sweeter and well worth the extra price because they are so much easier to digest. All milks are great sources of calcium, and at about the same price. Canned and powdered milks give you the most calcium for the price (and are great to keep on hand for cooking and baking), while fresh nonfat (also called skim), low-fat, and Lactaid® calcium-fortified nonfat give you the most calcium for the calories (300–625 mg/100 calories). Mix in a calcium-rich additive, like Carnation Instant Breakfast® or Alba Dairy Shake Mix®, and you've doubled your calcium in a single glass for under a dollar and fewer calories than a lowfat yogurt.

How about cheese? Well, there's news in that corner of the dairy case, too. As shown in Table 3, the reduced-fat and fat-free cheeses score high in amount of calcium for the calories (more than 300 mg/100 calories). Cottage cheese is a great source of protein and an important source of calcium (100–150 mg/100 calories for the traditional version, and 200 mg/100 calories for the calcium-fortified version). Yogurt is one of the most versatile dairy products, and, as reflected by the amount of refrigerator space it takes up in the supermarket, it's also one of the most popular. Yogurts range from nonfat plain, flavored, and fruited (fruit on the bottom or stirred), to low-fat plain, flavored, or fruited. More expensive per serving than milk or cheese, but a good nutritional buy in terms of calcium and a great breakfast, lunch, or snack, midafternoon or evening, yogurts provide about 350–400 mg of calcium per eight-ounce serving.

As I'm sure you've noticed by now, fat and calories are tied together, and the same food can have half the calories if the fat content has been reduced or eliminated. But we don't live by nutrition alone—let's not forget ice cream, an American tradition if there ever was one! While I would not advise looking to ice cream and frozen yogurt as your primary source of daily calcium, as shown in Table 4, even these treats can make an important contribution.

Calcium-fortified products, such as orange juice, are another alternative way to meet your calcium needs. Remember that the FDA

TABLE 3
Cheese and Yogurt Products

■ ■

Product	Amount	Calories	Fat (g)	Protein (g)	Calcium (mg)
Cheeses					
Regular cheddar	1.5 oz.	165	13.5	10.5	300
Reduced-fat cheddar	1.5 oz.	120	7.5	13.5	375
Lite cheddar	1.5 oz.	105	6	13.5	375
Fat-free cheddar	1.5 oz.	60	0	10	300
Cottage Cheese					
Nonfat	1/2 cup	70	0	13	100
Light n' Lively nonfat with calcium	1/2 cup	80	0	13	200
Light n' Lively lowfat with calcium	1/2 cup	80	1	12	200
2% fat	1/2 cup	90	2.5	13	80
4% fat	1/2 cup	110	4.5	13	100
Ricotta Cheese					
Regular	1/4 cup	90	6	7	150
Part-skim	1/4 cup	100	7	7	200
Light	1/4 cup	60	2.5	5	100
Low-fat	1/4 cup	60	2	9	300
Fat-free	1/4 cup	45	0	8	250
Yogurts					
Nonfat, flavored	8 oz.	100	0	9	350
Nonfat, fruited	8 oz.	100	0	9	350
Low-fat, flavored	8 oz.	210	3	10	400
Low-fat, fruited	8 oz.	240	3	9	350

ruling specifies that if a food is fortified with calcium, it must be in a form that is readily broken down and utilized by the body.[6] Depending on the brand you choose, in addition to being a great source of vitamin C, six ounces of calcium-fortified orange juice can give you 300–450 mg of calcium. If you choose this nontraditional

TABLE 4
Ice Cream and Frozen Yogurt Products

▪▪▪▪▪▪▪▪▪▪▪▪▪▪▪▪▪▪▪▪▪▪▪▪▪▪▪▪▪▪▪▪▪▪▪▪▪▪▪

Product	Amount	Calories	Fat (g)	Protein (g)	Calcium (mg)
Ice Cream					
Edy's Fat Free	1/2 cup	100	0	3	80
Kroger's Healthy Indulgence Fat Free	1/2 cup	50	0	3	100
Kroger's Healthy Indulgence Lowfat	1/2 cup	100	1.5	3	100
Kroger's Healthy Indulgence Premium Lowfat	1/2 cup	100	2	3	100
Breyer's Light Lowfat	1/2 cup	130	3	4	100
Kroger's Deluxe Lite	1/2 cup	110	3	2	100
Kroger's Deluxe Reduced Fat	1/2 cup	90	3.5	3	100
Breyer's Light	1/2 cup	130	4.5	3	100
Polar Pak	1/2 cup	120	7	2	40
Edy's Grand	1/2 cup	140	8	2	60
Breyer's	1/2 cup	160	10	4	100
Haagen-Dazs	1/2 cup	270	18	5	150
Frozen Yogurt					
Edy's Fat Free	1/2 cup	80	0	3	450
Breyer's Fat Free	1/2 cup	100	0	2	100
Polar Pak Low fat	1/2 cup	100	1.5	2	80
Edy's	1/2 cup	100	2.5	2	450

source of calcium in your daily diet, it's a good buy for the money and the calories (see Table 5).

In addition to dairy products and calcium-fortified orange juice, there are many other food sources of calcium, although they generally provide much less calcium per serving, or the calcium is present with binding agents that limit availability (e.g., spinach). Despite these limitations, these additional sources of calcium make important contributions to your daily diet (see Table 6).

TABLE 5
Regular and Calcium-Fortified Orange Juices

■ ■

Product	Amount	Calories	Fat (g)	Protein (g)	Calcium (mg)
Regular Orange Juice	6 oz.	150	0	1.5	0
Calcium-Fortified Orange Juices					
Kroger's 100% Orange Juice plus Calcium	6 oz.	150	0	3	300
Tropicana 100% Orange Juice plus Calcium	6 oz.	165	0	1	450
Minute Maid 100% Orange Juice with added Calcium	6 oz.	180	0	0	450

Designing Your Bone-Healthy Diet

Now that we have a better understanding of food sources of calcium and how to decipher nutrition information from the labels, let's look at how we can put this information to work in your daily diet. Shown in Table 7 are two menus, an original and a calcium-enriched version, based on the same or similar foods. As you can see, without adding either fat or calories, it's very simple to more than double the calcium content on an average day, just by careful food choices.

There are many other ways to easily incorporate calcium-rich foods into your daily diet, often lowering the fat content and making it healthier overall. To get you thinking bone-healthy, here are a few suggestions (the calcium contents are in parentheses). Bon appétit!

- For a vegetable side dish, substitute three-bean salad (120 mg/cup), spinach soufflé (250 mg/serving), or broccoli quiche (300 mg/serving).
- In soups, substitute evaporated nonfat milk (600 mg/cup) for cream (150 mg/cup).

TABLE 6
Nondairy Sources of Calcium
■■■

	Amount	Calories	Fat (g)	Protein (g)	Calcium (mg)
Fish and Seafood					
Sardines, including bones	1 oz.	50	3	6	92
Oysters, eastern, cooked	3 oz.	117	4	12	76
Salmon, including bones	3 oz.	118	5	17	180
Soybean Products					
Tofu, Soft Curd	1/2 cup	94	6	10	130
Tofu, Firm Curd	1/2 cup	183	11	20	260
Miso	1/2 cup	284	8	16	92
Natto	1/2 cup	187	10	15	190
Tempeh	1/2 cup	165	6	16	77
Fruits and Vegetables **(* indicates binding agents)**					
Spinach, boiled	1/2 cup	21	0	3	122*
Turnip Greens, boiled	1/2 cup	15	0	1	99*
Rhubarb, cooked and sweetened	1/2 cup	139	0	1	174*
Oranges	1 medium	65	0	1	60

- In cheesecakes, substitute nonfat ricotta (500 mg/cup).
- In omelets and salads, add grated, flaked, or crumbled hard cheese (200 mg/ounce).
- In cooking and baking, substitute chilled evaporated nonfat milk (600 mg/cup) for whipping cream (150 mg/cup).
- For salad dressing, try plain yogurt (400 mg/cup) seasoned with garlic, dry mustard, oregano, salt, and pepper.

TABLE 7

■■■■■■■■■■■■■■■■■■■■■■■■■■■■■■■■■■■■■■

Original Diet	Calcium-Enriched Diet	Calcium Improvement (mg)
Breakfast		
Orange juice	Orange juice with calcium	+450 mg
Bran cereal and nonfat milk	Bran cereal and calcium-fortified nonfat milk	+200 mg
Bagel with jelly	Bagel with reduced fat cheddar	+375 mg
Lunch		
Tuna salad sandwich	Salmon salad sandwich	+180 mg
Nonfat milk	Calcium-fortified nonfat milk	+200 mg
Fresh peach	Fresh orange	+60 mg
Dinner		
Beef stir-fry	Beef stir-fry with tofu (1/2 cup, firm curd)	+260 mg
Regular ice cream	Fat-free frozen yogurt	+350 mg
Total improvement		+2,075 mg

CHAPTER 11

Putting It All Together

A Game Plan for Action for Women of All Ages

Congratulations! You now have the knowledge to improve your own bone health and the bone health of your family, particularly your children and older relatives. In this chapter I'm going to pull together all of the risk factors I've discussed in the previous ten chapters and apply them in case studies. But first, let's summarize the seventeen risk factors for poor bone health in Table 1.

An individual with three or fewer risk factors (a Bone Health Risk Score of 3 or lower) is **low-risk.** A score of 4 is **moderate risk,** and a score of 5 or more is **high risk.**

Let's begin with Mary, from Chapter 1. She is probably our most extreme example of a woman at high risk for poor bone health, and at age 48, she has just been diagnosed with osteoporosis. Recall that Mary had been underweight for many years, had a late menarche (at age 16) and irregular menstrual periods, and had not been physically active in a long time. I've highlighted her risk factors in the list in Table 2. The Bone Health Risk Score is the total number of highlighted risk factors. With a Bone Health Risk Score of 6, Mary was at high risk for developing this disorder. At age 48, as she enters menopause, she faces an additional risk of being estrogen-deficient. Remember, there is a rapid loss of bone mass during those first few years around menopause, which would leave Mary with even poorer bone health and a greater risk of fractures in her later years.

In Chapter Two we met Emily and Lorraine. Remember that Emily was just beginning menopause, she had been physically active her whole life, has always had an adequate calcium intake, and has maintained a normal body weight and percent body fat. Her Bone Health Risk Score of 1, as shown in Table 3, tells us that she is at low risk for developing osteoporosis in her later years.

Lorraine, on the other hand, was underweight, was physically inactive, and had a poor calcium intake. Although they are sisters and they share a common genetic background, a lifetime of differences in several important health habits place them at opposite risks for developing osteoporosis at this stage in their lives. Lorraine's Bone Health Risk Score of 5 indicates that she is at high risk for poor bone health, and not surprisingly, she has already experienced several osteoporotic bone fractures.

TABLE 1

■■■■■■■■■■■■■■■■■■■■■■■■■■■■■■■■■

	Risk Categories	Risk Factors
Heredity Factors	Race	Asian or Caucasian
	Family history	+ Family history
Women-Only Factors	Age at menarche	Menarche at age 14 or older
	Menstrual cycles	Irregular
	Age at menopause	Menopause at age 45 or younger
	Total reproductive years	30 years or less
Body Shape Factors	Body build	Small-boned
	Proportion of fat to muscle	High fat/low muscle
	Weight	Underweight (BMI < 19.8)
Physical Factors	Exercise	Inactive
Prescription Factors	Hormonal status	Estrogen-deficient
	Certain medications	
Lifestyle Factors	Smoking	Smoker
	Alcohol	>one drink/day for women
		>two drinks/day for men
Nutrient Factors	Protein	High protein
	Sodium	High sodium
	Calcium	Low calcium
Bone Health Risk Score		

In Chapter Six we met Anna and Carrie. Anna is an 18-year-old ballerina, underweight for her height, and small-boned. She had not experienced menarche by age 18. Anna is Asian, and both her mother and grandmother have already been diagnosed with osteoporosis. Anna's Bone Health Risk Score of 6 (see Table 4) puts her

TABLE 2
Mary's Bone Health Risk Score
▪ ▪

Heredity Factors	Race	Asian or *Caucasian*
	– Family history	*+ Family history*
Women-Only Factors	Age at menarche	*Menarche at age 14 or older*
	Menstrual cycles	*Irregular*
	Age at menopause	Menopause at age 45 or younger
	Total reproductive years	30 years or less
Body Shape Factors	Body build	Small-boned
	Proportion of fat to muscle	High fat/low muscle
	Weight	*Underweight (BMI < 19.8)*
Physical Factors	Exercise	*Inactive*
Prescription Factors	Hormonal status	Estrogen-deficient
	Certain medications	
Lifestyle Factors	Smoking	Smoker
	Alcohol	>one drink/day for women
		>two drinks/day for men
Nutrient Factors	Protein	High protein
	Sodium	High sodium
	Calcium	Low calcium
Bone Health Risk Score		**6**

TABLE 3
▪▪▪▪▪▪▪▪▪▪▪▪▪▪▪▪▪▪▪▪▪▪▪▪▪▪▪▪▪▪▪▪

	Emily	*Lorraine*
Heredity Factors	Asian or *Caucasian*	Asian or *Caucasian*
	+ Family history	+ Family history
Women-Only Factors	Menarche at age	Menarche at age
	14 or older	14 or older
	Irregular	Irregular
	Menopause at age	Menopause at age
	45 or younger	45 or younger
	30 years or less	30 years or less
Body Shape Factors	Small-boned	Small-boned
	High fat/low muscle	*High fat/low muscle*
	Underweight	*Underweight*
	(BMI < 19.8)	*(BMI < 19.8)*
Physical Factors	Inactive	*Inactive*
Prescription Factors	Estrogen-deficient	Estrogen-deficient
	Certain medications	Certain medications
Lifestyle Factors	Smoker	Smoker
	>one drink/day for women	>one drink/day for women
	>two drinks/day for men	>two drinks/day for men
Nutrient Factors	High protein	High protein
	High sodium	High sodium
	Low calcium	*Low calcium*
Bone Health Risk Score	**1**	**5**

TABLE 4

▪ ▪

	Anna	*Carrie*
Heredity Factors	*Asian* or Caucasian	Asian or Caucasian
	+ Family history	+ Family history
Women-Only Factors	*Menarche at age*	Menarche at age
	14 or older	14 or older
	Irregular	Irregular
	Menopause at age	Menopause at age
	45 or younger	45 or younger
	30 years or less	30 years or less
Body Shape Factors	*Small-boned*	Small-boned
	High fat/low muscle	High fat/low muscle
	Underweight (BMI < 19.8)	Underweight (BMI < 19.8)
Physical Factors	Inactive	Inactive
Prescription Factors	*Estrogen-deficient*	Estrogen-deficient
	Certain medications	Certain medications
Lifestyle Factors	Smoker	Smoker
	>one drink/day for women	>one drink/day for women
	>two drinks/day for men	>two drinks/day for men
Nutrient Factors	High protein	*High protein*
	High sodium	*High sodium*
	Low calcium	Low calcium
Bone Health Risk Score	6	2

at high risk for developing osteoporosis, even now when she is still young. Carrie is 13-year-old gymnast who had taken a month off of training because of a sprained ankle. During that time her weight increased to a normal range for her height, and her periods began. Carrie is African-American. She likes milk, high-sodium snacks, and high-protein foods, but dislikes vegetables. Carrie's Bone Health Risk Score of 2 puts her at low risk, but there is still room for improvement.

There are several other girls and women I'd like you to meet. Jennifer is the oldest daughter of an Irish mother and an English father. At age 10, she was a chubby preteen with a solid build and big bones like her mother and grandmother. By age 12, she had grown six inches and gained 35 pounds. Her percent body fat had increased to 18% and her menstrual periods had begun. By age 14, she had grown another four inches to be 5'4" tall and gained another 30 pounds to be 135 pounds. Jennifer rarely participates in sports, preferring such leisure time activities as reading and going to the movies. She has begun smoking with her girlfriends, but hides it from her parents because she knows they will disapprove. Jennifer has a hardy appetite and loves dairy products. She drinks a quart of milk every day, and her favorite foods are pizza and cheesecake.

Allison is the youngest daughter of Chinese parents. At age 10, she began taking gymnastics in school. By age 12, she qualified for the State finals, and by age 14, she made the Olympic trials. She is small-boned, and she has grown into a graceful, slender adolescent. Between her demanding training schedule and the constant focus on maintaining a very trim physique, she has kept her weight to a minimum. At age 14, Allison is about 5", short for her age, weighs only 85 pounds, and has only 12% body fat. Her menstrual periods have not yet begun. Allison's grandmother died of complications of a hip fracture five years ago, and her mother has recently been diagnosed with osteoporosis. At home, Allison's mother cooks traditional Chinese foods, which Allison likes very much. At school, Allison eats mostly fruits and vegetables, and avoids meats and dairy products. As shown in Table 5, Jennifer's Bone Health Risk

TABLE 5
▪▪▪▪▪▪▪▪▪▪▪▪▪▪▪▪▪▪▪▪▪▪▪▪▪▪▪▪▪▪▪▪

	Jennifer	*Allison*
Heredity Factors	Asian or ***Caucasian***	***Asian*** or Caucasian
	+ Family history	***+ Family history***
Women-Only Factors	Menarche at age	***Menarche at age***
	14 or older	***14 or older***
	Irregular	Irregular
	Menopause at age	Menopause at age
	45 or younger	45 or younger
	30 years or less	30 years or less
Body Shape Factors	Small-boned	***Small-boned***
	High fat/low muscle	High fat/low muscle
	Underweight (BMI < 19.8)	***Underweight (BMI < 19.8)***
Physical Factors	**Inactive**	Inactive
Prescription Factors	Estrogen-deficient	Estrogen-deficient
	Certain medications	Certain medications
Lifestyle Factors	***Smoker***	Smoker
	>one drink/day for women	>one drink/day for women
	>two drinks/day for men	>two drinks/day for men
Nutrient Factors	High protein	High protein
	High sodium	***High sodium***
	Low calcium	***Low calcium***
Bone Health Risk Score	4	7

Score of 4 puts her at moderate risk, whereas Allison's score of 7 puts her at high risk, despite their young ages.

Margo is African-American. She has been an avid skater almost since she could walk. She was diagnosed with asthma about two years ago and takes corticosteroids by inhaler regularly. Her menstrual periods began when she was 12 years old. Margo has a medium build, and at age 15 she is 5'2" tall, weighs 105 pounds, and has 18% body fat. During one of her practices she fell and broke her leg when her two brothers crashed into her while they were playing ice hockey. She was on bedrest for two weeks. Margo's family is from the South, and her mother cooks traditional Southern food, which tends to be high in sodium.

Tammy, age 16, is of Northern European ancestry. Two years ago, Tammy was diagnosed with anorexia nervosa, an eating disorder characterized by an aversion to food and an obsession to become thin. She is currently receiving counseling through an adolescent psychiatric center. Small-boned, Tammy is 5'3" tall, weighs 90 pounds, and has 10% body fat. She has a family history of osteoporosis on both sides of her family. Tammy runs five miles every day, as well as doing an hour of aerobic exercises. She avoids all dairy products because she considers them fattening. Her menstrual periods have not yet begun. (See Table 6).

These girls illustrate important aspects of growth and development during adolescence, as well as the role of the major risk factors for poor bone health in the context of race, ethnicity, and family history. Fair-skinned individuals like Jennifer, Allison, and Tammy are at the greatest risk for developing osteoporosis. Margo's darker skin color and heavier muscles are a plus in her overall bone health. These girls also illustrate some of the additional risk factors for osteoporosis, such as smoking, illnesses, and medications. Teenage smoking is a major health problem in the United States. Nearly one out of four adult women in the United States is a smoker, and 90% began when they were teenagers. Smoking causes a spectrum of adverse health effects, including premature aging of the bones, by altering several bone-saving hormones. Margo's bone fracture and subsequent bedrest, as well as the corticosteroids she

TABLE 6
■■■■■■■■■■■■■■■■■■■■■■■■■■■■■■■

	Margo	*Tammy*
Heredity Factors	Asian or Caucasian	Asian or *Caucasian*
	+ Family history	+ *Family history*
Women-Only Factors	Menarche at age	*Menarche at age*
	14 or older	*14 or older*
	Irregular	Irregular
	Menopause at age	Menopause at age
	45 or younger	45 or younger
	30 years or less	30 years or less
Body Shape Factors	Small-boned	*Small-boned*
	High fat/low muscle	High fat/low muscle
	Underweight (BMI < 19.8)	*Underweight (BMI < 19.8)*
Physical Factors	*Inactive*	Inactive
Prescription Factors	Estrogen-deficient	Estrogen-deficient
	Certain medications	Certain medications
Lifestyle Factors	Smoker	Smoker
	>one drink/day for women	>one drink/day for women
	>two drinks/day for men	>two drinks/day for men
Nutrient Factors	High protein	High protein
	High sodium	High sodium
	Low calcium	*Low calcium*
Bone Health Risk Score	3	6

takes for her asthma, are additional risk factors for poor bone health. Tammy's anorexia nervosa is a major factor for her bone health; despite her regimen of physical activity, her bone health is suffering.

Hannah is 28 years old and pregnant for the first time. She was on oral contraceptives for about 10 years and stopped about six months ago. A gymnast in her teen years and a cheerleader in high school, she remains physically active in her adult years, walking to work every day and taking an exercise class twice a week. Hannah is of average build, weight, and percent body fat. An avid milk drinker, Hannah doesn't smoke or drink alcohol. Hannah is Caucasian, and her grandmother was hospitalized last year with a fractured hip.

Louise is 42 years old and is also pregnant for the first time. After ten years of recurring endometriosis, she underwent infertility treatments and conceived twins. Underweight for her height, Louise is small-boned. She rarely exercises, likes cheese and yogurt, and until she became pregnant, she had 2–3 glasses of wine with dinner every night. Louise was sent to a nutritionist by her obstetrician early in her pregnancy to help her plan her diet. Louise is also Caucasian, a nonsmoker, and has no family history of osteoporosis. Hannah's Bone Health Risk Score is 2, putting her at low risk, while Louise's score is 7, at high risk. Their risk factors are summarized in Table 7.

Although pregnancy itself is not a risk factor for poor bone health, the factors present both before and during this time in a woman's life can have an important influence on her later risk for osteoporosis. Hannah and Louise illustrate the extremes of these factors. Age is the single most important consideration for bone health: Louise is within a few years of entering menopause, while for Hannah it's probably more than 20 years away. And the years leading up to this pregnancy have been very different for each woman: Louise probably lost some bone mass with each treatment for endometriosis, while Hannah's bone mass was probably improved by her long-term use of oral contraceptives.

Although they both have included calcium-rich dairy products in their diets, Louise's lack of exercise and regular intake of alcohol, small bone size, low body weight, and lack of muscle as well as

TABLE 7

■■■■■■■■■■■■■■■■■■■■■■■■■■■■■■■■■■

	Hannah	*Louise*
Heredity Factors	Asian or *Caucasian*	Asian or *Caucasian*
	+ *Family history*	+ Family history
Women-Only Factors	Menarche at age	Menarche at age
	14 or older	14 or older
	Irregular	Irregular
	Menopause at age	Menopause at age
	45 or younger	45 or younger
	30 years or less	30 years or less
Body Shape Factors	Small-boned	*Small-boned*
	High fat/low muscle	*High fat/low muscle*
	Underweight (BMI < 19.8)	*Underweight (BMI < 19.8)*
Physical Factors	Inactive	*Inactive*
Prescription Factors	Estrogen-deficient	Estrogen-deficient
	Certain medications	*Certain medications*
Lifestyle Factors	Smoker	Smoker
	>one drink/day for women	*>one drink/day for women*
	>two drinks/day for men	>two drinks/day for men
Nutrient Factors	High protein	High protein
	High sodium	High sodium
	Low calcium	Low calcium
Bone Health Risk Score	2	7

her diagnosis of twins are all risk factors as she begins this pregnancy. Hannah's normal body weight and body fat, and lifelong habit of regular physical activity are factors in her favor. An adequate diet, with ample calcium, should help them both from losing ground during this pregnancy.

I hope these case studies have helped you put your own bone health risks into perspective. Score yourself, your daughter, your mother—see how bone-healthy your family is, and how you can improve those scores. I've included in the appendix a glossary of terms used throughout this book, as well as suggested additional readings and resources to help you have **Good Bones** for life.

References

Chapter Two: The Age Factor: The Most Important Factor

1. Rubinacci A, Sirtori P, Moro G, Galli L, Minoli I, Tessari L. Is there an impact of birth weight and early life nutrition on bone mineral content in preterm born infants and children? *Acta Paediatr* 1993; 82:711-3.

2. Bishop NJ, King FJ, Lucas A. Increased bone mineral content of preterm infants fed with a nutrient enriched formula after discharge from hospital. *Arch Dis Child* 1993; 68:573-8.

3. Schanler RJ, Burns PA, Abrams SA, Garza C. Bone mineralization in human milk fed preterm infants. *Pediatr Res* 1992; 31:583-6.

4. Pohlandt F. Prevention of postnatal bone demineralization in very low birth weight infants by individually monitored supplementation with calcium and phosphorus. *Pediatr Res* 1994; 35:125-9.

5. Chan GM. Growth and bone mineral status of discharged very low birth weight infants fed different formulas or human milk. *J Pediatr* 1993; 123:439-43.

6. Prestridge LL, Schanler RJ, Shulman RJ, Burns PA, Laine LL. Effect of parenteral calcium and phosphorus therapy on mineral retention and bone mineral content in very low birth weight infants. *J Pediatr* 1993; 122:761-8.

7. Minton S, Steichen J, Tsang R. Decreased bone mineral content in small for gestational infants compared with appropriate for gestational age infants. *Pediatrics* 1983; 71:383-8.

8. Petersen S, Gostfredsen A, Knudson F. Total body mineral content in light for gestational age infants and appropriate for gestational age infants. *Acta Paediatr Scand* 1989; 78:347-50.

9. Pohlandt F, Mathers N. Bone mineral content of appropriate and light for gestational age preterm and term newborn infants. *Acta Paediatr Scand* 1989; 78:835-9.

10. Namgung R, Tsang RC, Specker BL, Sierra RI, Ho ML. Reduced serum osteocalcin and 1,25-dihydroxyvitamin D concentrations and low bone mineral content in small for gestational age infants: Evidence of decreased bone formation rates. *J Pediatr* 1993; 122:269-75.

11. Namgung R, Tsang RC, Specker BL, Sierra RI, Ho ML. Low bone mineral content and high serum osteocalcin and 1,25-dihydroxyvitamin D in summer- versus winter-born newborn infants: An early fetal effect? *J Pediatr Gastroenterol Nutr* 1994; 19:220-7.

12. Del Rio L, Carrascosa A, Pons F, Gusinyé M, Yeste D, Domenech FM. Bone mineral density of the lumbar spine in white Mediterranean Spanish children and adolescents: Changes related to age, sex, and puberty. *Pediatr Res* 1994; 35:362-6.

13. Barrett-Connor E. The economics and human costs of osteoporotic fracture. *Am J Med* 1995; 98:3-5.

14. Chapuy MC, Arlot ME, Duboeuf F, et al. Vitamin D3 and calcium to prevent hip fractures in elderly women. *N Engl J Med* 1992; 327:1637-42.

15. Chevalley T, Rizzoli R, Nydegger V, et al. Effects of calcium supplements on femoral bone mineral density and vertebral fracture rate in vitamin D-replete elderly patients. *Osteoporos Int* 1994; 4:245-52.

16. Matkovic V, Kostial K, Simonovic I, et al. Bone status and fracture rates in two regions of Yugoslavia. *Am J Clin Nutr* 1979; 32:540-9.

17. Holbrook TL, Barrett-Connor E, Wingard DL. Dietary calcium and risk of hip fracture: 14-year prospective population study. *Lancet* 1988; 2:1046-9.

Chapter Three: The Heredity Factors: Race, Ethnicity, and Family History

1. Choi SC, Trotter M. A statistical study of the multivariate structure and race-sex differences of American white and negro fetal skeletons. *Am J Phys Anthropol* 1970; 33:307-12.

2. Trotter M, Peterson RR. Weight of the skeleton during postnatal development. *Am J Phys Anthropol* 1970; 33:313-24.

3. Griffin MR, Ray WA, Fought RL, Melton LJ. Black-white differences in fracture rates. *Am J Epidemiol* 1992; 136:1378-85.

4. Cummings SR, Kelsey JL, Nevitt MC, O'Dowd KJ. Epidemiology of osteoporosis and osteoporotic fractures. *Epidemiol Rev* 1985; 7:178-208.

5. Cohn SH, Abesamis C, Zanzi I, Aloia JF, Yasumura S, Ellis KJ. Body elemental composition: Comparison between black and white adults. *Am J Physiol* 1977; 232:E419-22.

6. Mulder H, Hackeng WHL, Silberbusch J. Racial differences in serum-calcitonin. *Lancet* 1979; 2:154.

7. Weinstein RS, Bell NH. Diminished rates of bone formation in normal black adults. *N Engl J Med* 1988; 319:1698-1701.

8. Bell NH, Yergey AL, Vieira NE, Oexmann MJ, Shary JR. Demonstration of a difference in urinary calcium, not calcium absorption, in black and white adolescents. *J Bone Miner Res* 1993; 8:1111-5.

9. Weinstein RS, Bell NH. Diminished rates of bone formation in normal black adults. *N Engl J Med* 1988; 319:1698-1701.

10. Cauley JA, Gutai JP, Kuller LH, Scott J, Nevitt MC. Black-white differences in serum sex hormones and bone mineral density. *Am J Epidemiol* 1994; 139:1035-46.

11. Harper AB, Laughlin WS, Mazess RB. Bone mineral content in St. Lawrence Island Eskimos. *Hum Biol* 1984; 56:63-78.

12. Mazess RB, Mather W. Bone mineral content of North Alaskan Esquimos. *Am J Clin Nutr* 1974; 27:916-25.

13. Nordin BEC. International patterns of osteoporosis. *Clin Orthop* 1966; 45:17-30.

14. Kahn SA, Pace JE, Cox ML, Gau DW, Cox SAL, Hodkinson HM. Osteoporosis and genetic influence: A three-generation study. *Postgrad Med J* 1994; 70:798-800.

15. Smith DM, Nance WE, Kang KW, Christian JC, Johnston CC. Genetic factor in determining bone mass. *J Clin Invest* 1973; 52:2800-8.

16. Dequeker J, Nijs J, Verstraeten A, Geusens P, Gevers G. Genetic determinants of bone mineral content at the spine and radius: A twin study. *Bone* 1987; 8:207-9.

17. Pocock AN, Eisman JA, Hopper JL, Yeates MG, Sambrook PN, Eberl S. Genetic determinants of bone mass in adults: A twin study. *J Clin Invest* 1987; 80:706-10.

18. Lutz J. Bone mineral, serum calcium, and dietary intake of mother/daughter pairs. *Am J Clin Nutr* 1986; 44:99-106.

19. Sowers MF, Burns TL, Wallace RB. Familial resemblance of bone mass in adult women. *Genet Epidemiol* 1986; 3:85-93.

20. McKay HA, Bailey DA, Wilkinson AA, Houston CS. Familial comparison of bone mineral density at the proximal femur and lumbar spine. *Bone Miner* 1994; 24:95-107.

21. Seeman E, Hopper JL, Bach LA, Cooper ME, Parkinson E, McKay J, Jerums G. Reduced bone mass in daughters of women with osteoporosis. *N Engl J Med* 1989; 320:554-8.

22. Lutz J, Tesar R. Mother-daughter pairs: Spinal and femoral bone densities and dietary intakes. *Am J Clin Nutr* 1990; 52:872-7.

23. Jouanny P, Guillemin F, Kuntz C, Jeandel C, Pourel J. Environmental and genetic factors affecting bone mass: Similarity of bone density among members of healthy families. *Arthritis Rheum* 1995; 38:61-7.

24. Slemenda CW, Christian JC, Williams CJ, Norton JA, Johnston CC. Genetic determinants of bone mass in adult women: A reevaluation of the twin model and the potential importance of gene interaction on heritability estimates. *J Bone Miner Res* 1991; 6:561-7.

25. Morrison NA, Qi JC, Tokita A, et al. Prediction of bone density from vitamin D receptor alleles. *Nature* 1994; 367:284-7.

Chapter Four: The Women-Only Factors: From Menarche to Menopause

1. Meyer F, Moisan J, Marcoux D, Bouchard C. Dietary and physical determinants of menarche. *Epidemiol* 1990; 1:377-81.

2. Frisch RE, McArthur JW. Menstrual cycles: Fatness as a determinant of minimum weight for height necessary for their maintenance or onset. *Science* 1974; 185:949-50.

3. Cooper GS, Sandler DP. Long-term effects of reproductive-age menstrual cycle patterns on peri- and postmenopausal fracture risk. *Am J Epidemiol* 1997; 145:804-9.

4. Johnell O, Nilsson BE. Life-style and bone mineral mass in perimenopausal women. *Calcif Tissue Int* 1984; 36:354-6.

5. Fox KM, Magaziner J, Sherwin R, et al. Reproductive correlates of bone mass in elderly women. *J Bone Miner Res* 1993; 8:901-8.

6. Paganinini-Hill A, Chao A, Ross RK, et al. Exercise and other factors in the prevention of hip fracture: the Leisure World Study. *Epidemiology* 1991; 2:16-25.

7. Warren MP, Brooks-Gunn J, Fox RP, Lancelot C, Newman D, Hamilton WG. Lack of bone accretion and amenorrhea: Evidence for a relative osteopenia in weight-bearing bones. *J Clin Endocrinol Metab* 1991; 72:847-853.

8. Cann CE, Martin MC, Jaffee RB. Duration of amenorrhea affects rate of bone loss in women runners: Implications for therapy. *Med Sci Sports Exerc* 1985; 17:214-9.

9. Jonnavithula S, Warren MP, Fox RP, Lazaro MI. Bone density is compromised in amenorrheic women despite return of menses: A 2-year study. *Obstet Gynecol* 1993; 81:669-74.

10. Cann CE, Cavanagh DJ, Schnurpfiel K, Martin MC. Menstrual history is the primary determinant of trabecular bone density in women. *Med Sci Sports Exerc* 1988; 20 (Suppl 2):S59 Abs.

11. Committee on Gynecologic Practice. Estrogen dose in oral contraceptives. American College of Obstetricians and Gynecologists committee opinion, number 60, March 1988, Reaffirmed, 1991.

12. Rosenberg L, Palmer JR, Zauber AG, et al. A case-control study of oral contraceptive use and invasive epithelial ovarian cancer. *Am J Epidemiol* 1994; 139:654-61.

13. Gross TP, Schlesselman JJ. The estimated effect of oral contraceptive use on the cumulative risk of epithelial ovarian cancer. *Obstet Gynecol* 1994; 83:419-24.

14. Schlesselman JJ. Net effect of oral contraceptive use on the risk of cancer in women in the United States. *Obstet Gynecol* 1995; 85:793-801.

15. Petitti DB, Sidney S, Bernstein A, Wolf S, Quesenberry C, Ziel HK. Stroke in users of low-dose oral contraceptives. *N Engl J Med* 1996; 335:8-15.

16. Corson SL. Oral contraceptives for the prevention of osteoporosis. *J Reprod Med* 1993; 38:1015-20.

17. Lindsay R, Tohme J, Kanders B. The effect of oral contraceptive use on vertebral bone mass in pre- and post-menopausal women. *Contraception* 1986; 34:333-40.

18. Stevenson J, Lees B, Davenport M, et al. Determinants of bone density in normal women: Risk factors for future osteoporosis. *Br Med J* 1989; 298:924-8.

19. Recker RR, Davies KM, Hinders SM, et al. Bone gain in young adult women. *JAMA* 1992; 268:2403-8.

20. DeCherney A. Bone-sparing properties of oral contraceptives. *Am J Obstet Gynecol* 1996; 174:15-20.

21. Hergenroeder AC, Smith EOB, Shypailo R, Jones LA, Klish WJ, Ellis K. Bone mineral changes in young women with hypothalamic amenorrhea treated with oral contraceptives, medroxyprogesterone, or placebo over 12 months. *Am J Obstet Gynecol* 1997; 176:1017-25.

22. Kitai E, Blum M, Kaplan B. The bone sparing effect of oral contraceptive use in non-smoking women. *Clin Exp Obstet Gyn* 1992; 19:30-3.

23. Kritz-Silverstein D, Barrett-Connor E. Bone mineral density in postmenopausal women as determined by prior oral contraceptive use. *Am J Public Health* 1993; 83:100-2.

24. Kleerekoper M, Brienza RS, Schultz LR, et al. Oral contraceptive use may protect against low bone mass. *Arch Intern Med* 1991; 151:1971-6.

25. Orwoll ES, Yuzpe AA, Burry KA, et al. Nafarelin therapy in endometriosis: Long-term effects on bone mineral density. *Am J Obstet Gynecol* 1994; 171:1221-5.

26. Elred JM, Haynes PJ, Thomas EJ. A randomized double blind placebo controlled trial of the effects on bone metabolism of the combination of nafarelin acetate and norethisterone. *Clin Endocrinol* 1992; 37:354-9.

27. Dawood MY. Impact of medical treatment of endometriosis on bone mass. *Am J Obstet Gynecol* 1993; 168:674-84.

28. Lane N, Baptista J, Snow-Harter C. Bone mineral density of the lumbar spine in endometriosis subjects compared to an age-similar control population. *J Clin Endocrinol Metab* 1991; 72:510-4.

29. Gambacciani M, Spinetti A, Gallo R, et al. Ultrasonographic bone characteristics during normal pregnancy: Longitudinal and cross-sectional evaluation. *Am J Obstet Gynecol* 1995; 173:890-3.

30. Okah FA, Tsang RC, Sierra R, Brady KK, Specker BL. Bone turnover and mineral metabolism in the last trimester of pregnancy: Effect of multiple gestation. *Obstet Gynecol* 1996; 88:168-73.

31. Simon JA, Browner WS, Tao JL, Hulley SB. Calcium intake and blood pressure in elderly women. *Am J Epidemiol* 1992; 136:1241-7.

32. Iso H, Kitamura A, Sato S, et al. Calcium intake and blood pressure in seven Japanese populations. *Am J Epidemiol* 1991; 133:776-83.

33. Kynast-Gales SA, Massey LK. Effects of dietary calcium from dairy products on ambulatory blood pressure in hypertensive men. *J Am Diet Assoc* 1992; 92:1497-501.

34. Osborne CG, McTyre RB, Dudek J, et al. Evidence for the relationship of calcium to blood pressure. *Nutr Rev* 1996; 54:365-81.

35. Bucher HC, Cook RJ, Guyatt GH, et al. Effects of dietary calcium supplementation on blood pressure: A meta-analysis of randomized controlled trials. *JAMA* 1996; 275:1016-22.

36. Repke JT, Villar J, Anderson C, et al. Biochemical changes associated with blood pressure reduction induced by calcium supplementation during pregnancy. *Am J Obstet Gynecol* 1989; 160:684-90.

37. Villar J, Repke JT. Calcium supplementation during pregnancy may reduce preterm delivery in high-risk populations. *Am J Obstet Gynecol* 1990; 163:1124-31.

38. Belizan JM, Villar J, Gonzalez L, Campodonico L, Bergel E. Calcium supplementation to prevent hypertensive disorders of pregnancy. *N Engl J Med* 1991; 325:1399-405.

39. Repke JT, Villar J. Pregnancy-induced hypertension and low birth weight: The role of calcium. *Am J Clin Nutr* 1991; 54:237S-41S.

40. Marcoux S, Brisson J, Fabia J. Calcium intake from dairy products and supplements and the risks of preeclampsia and gestational hypertension. *Am J Epidemiol* 1991; 133:1266-72.

41. Richardson BE, Baird DD. A study of milk and calcium supplement intake and subsequent preeclampsia in a cohort of pregnant women. *Am J Epidemiol* 1995; 141:667-73.

42. Hayslip CC, Klein TA, Wray HL, Duncan WE. The effects of lactation on bone mineral content in healthy postpartum women. *Obstet Gynecol* 1989; 73:588-92.

43. Specker BL, Tsang RC, Ho ML. Changes in calcium homeostasis over the first year postpartum: Effect of lactation and weaning. *Obstet Gynecol* 1991; 78:56-62.

44. Sowers MF, Corton G, Shapiro B, et al. Changes in bone density with lactation. *JAMA* 1993; 269:3130-5.

45. Sowers MF, Randolph J, Shapiro B, Jannausch M. A prospective study of bone density and pregnancy after an extended period of lactation with bone loss. *Obstet Gynecol* 1995; 85:285-9.

46. Kalkwarf HJ, Specker BL. Bone mineral loss during lactation and recovery after weaning. *Obstet Gynecol* 1995; 86:26-32.

47. Krebs NF, Reidinger CJ, Robertson AD, Brenner M. Bone mineral changes during lactation: Maternal, dietary, and biochemical correlates. *Am J Clin Nutr* 1997; 65:1738-46.

48. Kalkwarf HJ, Specker BL, Bianchi DC, Ranz J, Ho M. The effect of calcium supplementation on bone density during lactation and after weaning. *N Engl J Med* 1997; 337:523-8.

49. Watson NR, Studd JWW, Garnett T, Savvas M, Milligan P. Bone loss after hysterectomy with ovarian conservation. *Obstet Gynecol* 1995; 86:72-7.

50. Riedel HH, Lehmann-Willenbrock A, Semm K. Ovarian failure phenomena after hysterectomy. *J Reprod Med* 1986; 31:597-600.

51. Siddle N, Sarrel P, Whitehead M. The effect of hysterectomy on the age at ovarian failure: Idenitification of a subgroup of women with premature loss of ovarian function and literiture review. *Fertil Steril* 1987; 47:94-100.

52. Stone SC, Dickey RP, Mickal A. The acute effect of hysterectomy on ovarian function. *Am J Obstet Gynecol* 1975; 121:193-7.

53. Georgiou E, Ntalles K, Papageorgiou A, et al. Bone mineral loss related to menstrual history. *Acta Orthop Scand* 1989; 60:192-4.

54. Barzel US. Estrogens in the prevention and treatment of postmenopausal osteoporosis: A review. *Am J Med* 1988; 85:847-9.

55. Elders PJM, Netelenbos JC, Lips P, et al. Perimenopausal bone mass and risk factors. *Bone Miner* 1989; 7:289-99.

56. Gardsell P, Johnell O, Nilsson BE. The impact of menopausal age on future fragility fracture risk. *J Bone Miner Res* 1991; 6:429-33.

57. Richelson LS, Wahner HW, Melton LJ III, Riggs BL. Relative contributions of aging and estrogen deficiency to postmenopausal bone loss. *N Engl J Med* 1984; 311:1273-5.

58. Parazzini F, Bidoli E, Franceschi S, et al. Menopause, menstrual and reproductive history, and bone mineral density in northern Italy. *J Epidemiol Community Health* 1996; 50:519-23.

59. Kritz-Silverstein D, Barrett-Connor E. Early menopause, number of reproductive years, and bone mineral density in postmenopausal women. *Am J Public Health* 1993; 83:983-8.

60. Melton LJ III, Bryant SC, Wahner HW, et al. Influence of breastfeeding and other reproductive factors on bone mass later in life. *Osteoporos Int* 1993; 3:76-83.

61. Vico L, Prallet B, Chappard D, Alexandre C. Lumbar bone density and reproductive years. *J Bone Miner Res* 1991; 6 (Suppl 1):S162. Abstract.

Chapter Five: The Body Shape Factors: Muscle, Fat, and Body Weight

1. Sowers MFR, Kshirsagar A, Crutchfield MM, Updike S. Joint influence of fat and lean body composition compartments on femoral bone mineral density in premenopausal women. *Am J Epidemiol* 1992; 136:257-65.

2. Ulrich CM, Georgiou CC, Snow-Harter CM, Gilles DE. Bone mineral density in mother-daughter pairs: Relations to lifetime exercise, lifetime milk consumption, and calcium supplements. *Am J Clin Nutr* 1996; 63:72-9.

3. Slemenda CW, Reister TK, Hui SL, Miller JZ, Christian JC, Johnston CC. Influences on skeletal mineralization in children and adolescents: Evidence for varying effects of sexual maturation and physical activity. *J Pediatr* 1994; 125:201-7.

4. Rubin K, Schirduan V, Gendreau P, Sarfarazi M, Mendola R, Dalsky G. Predictors of axial and peripheral bone mineral density in healthy children and adolescents, with special attention to the role of puberty. *J Pediatr* 1993; 123:863-70.

5. Gordon CL, Webber CE. Body composition and bone mineral distribution during growth in females. *J Assoc Can Radiol* 1993; 44:112-6.

6. Miller JZ, Slemenda CW, Meaney FJ, Reister TK, Hui S, Johnston CC. The relationship of bone mineral density and anthropometric variables in healthy male and female children. *Bone Miner* 1991; 14:137-52.

7. Mora S, Goodman WG, Loro ML, Roe TF, Sayre J, Gilsanz V. Age-related changes in cortical and cancellous vertebral bone density in girls: Assessment with quantitative CT. *Am J Radiol* 1994; 162:405-9.

8. Turner JG, Gilchrist NL, Ayling EM, Hassall AJ, Hooke EA, Sadler WA. Factors affecting bone mineral density in high school girls. *N Z Med J* 1992; 105:95-6.

9. Prevalence of overweight among adolescents—United States, 1988-91. *Morb Mortal Weekly Report* 1994; 43:818-21.

10. Update: Prevalence of overweight among children, adolescents, and adults—United States, 1988-1994. *Morb Mortal Weekly Report* 1997; 46:199-202.

11. Guo SS, Roche AF, Chumlea WC, Gardner JD, Siervogel RM. The predictive value of childhood body mass index values for overweight at age 35 y. *Am J Clin Nutr* 1994; 59:810-9.

12. Kolata G. Obese children: A growing problem. *Science* 1986; 232:20-1.

13. Simon JA, Morrison JA, Similo SL, McMahon RP, Schreiber GB. Correlates of high-density lipoprotein cholesterol in black girls and white girls: The NHLBI growth and health study. *Am J Public Health* 1995; 85:1698-702.

14. Hager RL, Tucker LA, Seljaas GT. Aerobic fitness, blood lipids, and body fat in children. *Am J Public Health* 1995; 85:1702-6.

15. Committee on Sports Medicine and Fitness. Fitness, activity, and sports participation in the preschool child. *Pediatrics* 1992; 90:1002-4.

16. US Dept Health Human Services. *1985 President's Council on Physical Fitness and Sports Youth Fitness Survey.* Washington, DC: US Govt. Printing Office, 1986.

17. Bachrach LK, Katzman DK, Litt IF, Guido D, Marcus R. Recovery from osteopenia in adolescent girls with anorexia nervosa. *J Clin Endocrinol Metab* 1991; 72:602-6.

18. Kiriike N, Iketani KN, Nakanishi S, et al. Reduced bone density and major hormones regulating calcium metabolism in anorexia nervosa. *Acta Psychiatr Scand* 1992; 86:358-63.

19. Abrams SA, Silber TJ, Esteban NV, et al. Mineral balance and bone turnover in adolescents with anorexia nervosa. *J Pediatr* 1993; 123:326-31.

20. Kuczmarski RJ, Flegal KM, Campbell SM, Johnson CL. Increasing prevalence of overweight among US adults: The National Health and Nutrition Examination Surveys, 1960 to 1991. *JAMA* 1994; 272:205-11.

21. Kritz-Silverman D, Barrett-Connor E. Long-term postmenopausal hormone use, obesity, and fat distribution in older women. *JAMA* 1996; 275:46-9.

22. Aloia JF, Vaswani A, Russo L, Sheehan M, Flaster E. The influence of menopause and hormonal replacement therapy on body cell mass and body fat mass. *Am J Obstet Gynecol* 1995; 172:896-900.

23. Wang Q, Hassager C, Ravn P, Wang S, Christiansen C. Total and regional body-composition changes in early postmenopausal women:Age-related or menopause related? *Am J Clin Nutr* 1994; 60:843-8.

24. Ito M, Hayashi K, Uetani M, Yamada M, Ohki M, Nakamura T. Association between anthropometric measures and spinal bone mineral density. *Invest Radiol* 1994; 29:812-6.

25. Rico H, Revilla M, Villa LF, Alvarez del Buergo M, Ruiz-Contreras D. Determinants of total-body and regional bone mineral content and density in postpubertal normal women. *Metabolism* 1994; 43:263-6.

26. Kahn HS, Tatham LM, Rodriguez C, Calle EE, Thun MJ, Heath CW. Stable behaviors associated with adults' 10-year change in body mass index and likelihood of gain at the waist. *Am J Public Health* 1997; 87:747-54.

Chapter Six: The Physical Factors: Exercise and Physical Activity

1. Chalmers J, Ho KC. Geographic variations in senile osteoporosis:The association with physical activity. *J Bone Joint Surg* 1970; 52B:667-75.

2. Lees B, Molleson T, Arnett TR, Stevenson JC. Differences in proximal femur bone density over two centuries. *Lancet* 1993; 1:673-5.

3. Slemenda CW, Miller JZ, Hui SL, Reister TK, Johnson CC. Role of physical activity in the development of skeletal mass in children. *J Bone Miner Res* 1991; 6:1227-33.

4. Telama R, Yang X, Laakso L, Viikari J. Physical activity in childhood and adolescence as predictor of physical activity in young adulthood. *Am J Prev Med* 1997; 13:317-23.

5. Haliova L, Anderson JJB. Lifetime calcium intake and physical activity habits:Independent and combined effects on the radial bone of healthy premenopausal women. *Am J Clin Nutr* 1989; 49:534-41.

6. Greendale GA, Barrett-Connor E, Edelstein S, Ingles S, Haile R. Lifetime leisure exercise and osteoporosis: The Rancho Bernardo study. *Am J Epidemiol* 1995; 141:951-9.

7. Jaglal SB, Kreiger N, Darlington G. Past and recent physical activity and risk of hip fracture. *Am J Epidemiol* 1993; 138:107-18.

8. Female athlete triad risk for women. *JAMA* 1993; 270:921-3.

9. Tofler IR, Stryer BK, Micheli LJ, Herman LR. Physical and emotional problems of elite female gymnasts. *N Engl J Med* 1996; 335:281-3.

10. Warren MP, Brooks-Gunn J, Hamilton LH, Warren LF, Hamilton WG. Scoliosis and fractures in young ballet dancers. *N Engl J Med* 1986; 314:1348-53.

11. Warren MP, Brooks-Gunn J, Fox RP, Lancelot C, Newman D, Hamilton WG. Lack of bone accretion and amenorrhea: Evidence for a relative osteopenia in weight-bearing bones. *J Clin Endocrinol Metab* 1991; 72:847-53.

12. Frisch RE, Wyshak G, Vincent L. Delayed menarche and amenorrhea in ballet dancers. *N Engl J Med* 1980; 303:17-19.

13. Young N, Formica C, Szmukler G. Bone density at weight-bearing and nonweight-bearing sites in ballet dancers: The effects of exercise, hypogonadism, and body weight. *J Clin Endocrinol Metab* 1994; 78:449-54.

14. Drinkwater BL, Nilson K, Chesnut CH, Bremner WJ, Shainholtz S, Southworth MB. Bone mineral content of amenorrheic and eumenorrheic athletes. *N Engl J Med* 1984; 311:277-81.

15. Wolman RL, Clark P, McNally E, Harries MG, Reeve J. Dietary calcium as a statistical determinant of spinal trabecular bone density in amenorrhoeic and oestrogen-replete athletes. *Bone Miner* 1992; 17:415-23.

16. Rencken ML, Chesnut CH, Drinkwater BL. Bone density at multiple skeletal sites in amenorrheic athletes. *JAMA* 1996; 276:238-40.

17. Fischer EC, Nelson ME, Frontera WR, Turksoy RN, Evans WJ. Bone mineral content and levels of gonadotropins and estrogens in amenorrheic running women. *J Clin Endocrinol Metab* 1986; 62:1232-6.

18. Lindberg JS, Fears WB, Hunt MM, Powell MR, Boll D, Wade CE. Exercise-induced amenorrhea and bone density. *Ann Intern Med* 1984; 101:647-8.

19. Snead DB, Stubbs CC, Weltman JY, et al. Dietary patterns, eating behaviors, and bone mineral density in women runners. *Am J Clin Nutr* 1992; 56:705-11.

20. Louis O, Demeirleir K, Kalender W, et al. Low vertebral bone density values in young non-elite female runners. *Int J Sports Med* 1991; 12:214-7.

21. Nelson ME, Fisher EC, Catsos PD, Meredith CN, Turksoy RN, Evans WJ. Diet and bone status in amenorrheic runners. *Am J Clin Nutr* 1986; 43:910-6.

22. Baer JT, Taper LJ, Gwazdauskas FG, et al. Diet, hormonal, and metabolic factors affecting bone mineral density in adolescent amenorrheic and eumenorrheic female runners. *J Sports Med Phys Fitness* 1992; 32:51-8.

23. Jonnavithula S, Warren MP, Fox RP, Lazaro MI. Bone density is compromised in amenorrheic women despite return of menses: A 2-year study. *Obstet Gynecol* 1993; 81:669-74.

24. Drinkwater BL, Bruemner B, Chesnut CH. Menstrual history as a determinant of current bone density in young athletes. *JAMA* 1990; 263:545-8.

25. Rico H, Revilla M, Villa LF, Gómez-Castresana F, Alvarez del Buergo M. Body composition in postpubertal boy cyclists. *J Sports Med Phys Fitness* 1993; 33:278-81.

26. Smith R, Rutherford OM. Spine and total body bone mineral density and serum testosterone levels in male athletes. *Eur J Appl Physiol* 1993; 67:330-4.

27. Theintz GE, Howald H, Weiss U, Sizonenko PC. Evidence for a reduction of growth potential in adolescent female gymnasts. *J Pediatr* 1993; 122:306-13.

28. Meeusen R, Borms J. Gymnastic injuries. *Sports Med* 1992; 13:337-56.

29. Mansfield MJ, Emans SJ. Growth in female gymnasts: Should training decrease during puberty? *J Pediatr* 1993; 122:237-9.

30. Slemenda CW, Johnston CC. High intensity activities in young women: Site specific bone mass effects among female figure skaters. *Bone Miner* 1993; 20:125-32.

31. Conroy BP, Kraemer WJ, Maresh CM, et al. Bone mineral density in elite junior Olympic weightlifters. *Med Sci Sports Exerc* 1993; 25:1103-9.

32. Karlsson MK, Johnell O, Obrant KJ. Bone mineral density in weight lifters. *Calcif Tissue Int* 1993; 52:212-5.

33. Jacobson PC, Beaver C, Grubb SA, Taft TN, Talmage RV. Bone density in women: College athletes and older athletic women. *J Orthop Res* 1984; 2:328-32.

34. Krahl H, Michaelis U, Pieper H-G, Quack G, Montag M. Stimulation of bone growth through sports: A radiologic investigation of the upper extremities in professional tennis players. *Am J Sports Med* 1994; 22:751-7.

35. Haapasalo H, Kannus P, Sievänen H, Heinonen A, Oja P, Vuori I. Long-term unilateral loading and bone mineral density and content in female squash players. *Calcif Tissue* 1994; 54:249-55.

36. Taaffe DR, Snow-Harter C, Connolly DA, Robinson TL, Brown MD, Marcus R. Differential effects of swimming versus weight-bearing activity on bone mineral status of eumenorrheic athletes. *J Bone Miner Res* 1995; 10:586-93.

37. Grimston SK, Willows ND, Hanley DA. Mechanical loading regime and its relationship to bone mineral density in children. *Med Sci Sports Exerc* 1993; 25:1203-10.

38. McCulloch RC, Bailey DA, Houston CS, Dodd BL. Effects of physical activity, dietary calcium intake, and selected lifestyle factors on bone density in young women. *Can Med Assoc J* 1990; 142:221-7.

39. Metz JA, Anderson JJB, Gallagher PN. Intakes of calcium, phosphorus, and protein, and physical activity level are related to radial bone mass in young adult women. *Am J Clin Nutr* 1993; 58:537-42.

40. Welten DC, Kemper HCG, Post GB, et al. Weight-bearing activity during youth is a more important factor for peak bone mass than calcium intake. *J Bone Miner Res* 1994; 9:1089-96.

41. Kriska AM, Sandler RB, Cauley JA, LaPorte RE, Hom DL, Pambianco G. The assessment of historical physical activity and its relation to adult bone parameters. *Am J Epidemiol* 1988; 127:1053-61.

42. Schoutens A, Laurent E, Poortmans JR. Effects of inactivity and exercise on bone. *Sports Med* 1989; 7:71-81.

43. Snow-Harter C, Marcus R. Exercise, bone mineral density, and osteoporosis. *Exerc Sport Sci Rev* 1991; 19:351-88.

44. Anderson JJB, Tylavsky FA, Lacey JM, Talmage RV, Taft T. Major factors influencing distal radial bone mass in college-age women. *Fed Proc* 1987; 46:632 (abstr).

45. Hahn RA, Teutsch SM, Rothenberg RB, Marks JS. Excess deaths from nine chronic diseases in the United States. *JAMA* 1986; 264:2654-9.

46. McGinnis JM, Foege WH. Actual causes of death in the United States. *JAMA* 1993; 270:2207-12.

47. Monthly estimates of leisure-time physical inactivity—United States, 1994. *Morb Mortal Weekly Rep* 1997; 46:393-7.

48. Simon JA, Morrison JA, Similo SL, McMahon RP, Schreiber GB. Correlates of high-density lipoprotein cholesterol in black girls and white girls: the NHLBI growth and health study. *Am J Public Health* 1995; 85:1698-702.

49. Pate RR, Pratt M, Blair SN, et al. Physical activity and public health: A recommendation from the Centers for Disease Control and Prevention and the American College of Sports Medicine. *JAMA* 1995; 273:402-7.

50. Fletcher GF, Balady G, Froelicher VF, Hartley LH, Haskell WL, Pollock ML. Exercise standards: A statement for healthcare professionals from the American Heart Association. *Circulation* 1995; 91:580-615.

Chapter Seven: The Prescription Factor: Hormones, Medications, and Supplements

1. American College of Obstetricians and Gynecologists. Hormone replacement therapy. *ACOG Technical Bulletin,* Number 166—April, 1992.

2. Tepper R, Goldberger S, May JY, Luz IJ, Beyth Y. Hormonal replacement therapy in postmenopausal women and cardiovascular disease: An overview. *Obstet Gynecol Surv* 1992; 47:426-31.

3. Udoff L, Langenberg P, Adashi EY. Combined continuous hormone replacement therapy: A critical review. *Obstet Gynecol* 1995; 86:306-16.

4. Speroff L, Rowan J, Symons J, et al. The comparative effect on bone density, endometrium, and lipids of continuous hormones as replacement therapy (the CHART study). *JAMA* 1996; 276:1397-403.

5. Wild RA. Estrogen: Effects on the cardiovascular tree. *Obstet Gynecol* 1996; 87: 27S-35S.

6. Kanis JA, Melton LJ, Christiansen C, Johnston CC, Khaltaev N. The diagnosis of osteoporosis. *J Bone Miner Res* 1994; 9:1137-141.

7. Cummings SR, Black DM, Nevitt MC, et al. Bone density at various sites for prediction of hip fractures. *Lancet* 1993; 341:72-5.

8. Heaney RP. Bone mass, nutrition, and other lifestyle factors. *Nutr Rev* 1996; 54: S3-S10.

9. Schneider DL, Barrett-Connor EL, Morton DJ. Timing of postmenopausal estrogen for optimal bone mineral density. *JAMA* 1997; 277:543-7.

10. The Writing Group for the PEPI Trial. Effects of hormone therapy on bone mineral density: Results from the Postmenopausal Estrogen/Progestin Intervention (PEPI) Trial. *JAMA* 1996; 276:1389-96.

11. Grady D, Gebretsadik T, Kerlikowske K, Ernster V, Petitti D. Hormone replacement therapy and endometrial cancer risk: A meta-analysis. *Obstet Gynecol* 1995; 85:304-13.

12. Stanford JL, Weiss NS, Voigt LF, Daling JR, Habel LA, Rossing MA. Combined estrogen and progestin hormone replacement therapy in relation to risk of breast cancer in middle-aged women. *JAMA* 1995; 274:137-42.

13. Adami H-O, Persson I. Hormone replacement and breast cancer: A remaining controversy? (Editorial). *JAMA* 1995; 274:178-9.

14. Speroff L. Postmenopausal hormone therapy and breast cancer. *Obstet Gynecol* 1996; 87:44S-54S.

15. Cummings SR, Black DM, Rubin SM. Lifetime risks of hip, Colles', or vertebral fracture and coronary heart disease among white postmenopausal women. *Arch Intern Med* 1989; 149:2445-8.

16. Brinton LA, Schairer C. Postmenopausal hormone-replacement therapy—Time for reappraisal? (Editorial). *N Engl J Med* 1997; 336:1821-2.

17. Gorsky RD, Koplan JP, Peterson HB, Thacker SB. Relative risks and benefits of long-term estrogen replacement therapy: A decision analysis. *Obstet Gynecol* 1994; 83:161-6.

18. Liberman UA, Weiss SR, Bröll J, et al. Effect of oral alendronate on bone mineral density and the incidence of fractures in postmenopausal osteoporosis. *N Engl J Med* 1995; 333:1437-43.

19. Black DM, Cummings SR, Karpf DB, et al. Randomized trial of alendronate on risk of fracture in women with existing vertebral fractures. *Lancet* 1996; 2:1535-41.

20. Karpf DB, Shapiro DR, Seeman E, et al. Prevention of nonvertebral fractures by alendronate: A meta-analysis. *JAMA* 1997; 277:1159-64.

21. McIntyre I, Whitehead MI, Banks LM, Stevenson JC, Wimalawansa SJ, Healy MJR. Calcitonin for prevention of postmenopausal bone loss. *Lancet* 1988; 1:900-2.

22. Tiegs RD, Body JJ, Wahner HW, et al. Calcitonin secretion in postmenopausal osteoporosis. *N Engl J Med* 1985; 312:1097-1100.

23. Ellerington MC, Hillard TC, Whitcroft SIJ, et al. Intranasal salmon calcitonin for the prevention and treatment of postmenopausal osteoporosis. *Calcif Tissue Int* 1996; 59:6-11.

24. Pak CY, Sakhaee K, Zerwekh JE, Parcel C, Peterson R, Johnson K. Safe and effective treatment of osteoporosis with intermittent slow-release sodium fluoride: Augmentation of vertebral bone mass and inhibition of fractures. *J Clin Endocrinol Metab* 1989; 68:150-9.

25. Pak CY, Sakhaee K, Piziak V, et al. Slow-release sodium fluoride in the management of postmenopausal osteoporosis. *Ann Intern Med* 1994; 120:625-32.

26. Pak CYC, Sakhaee K, Adams-Huet B, Piziak V, Peterson RD, Poindexter JR. Treatment of postmenopausal osteoporosis with slow-release sodium fluoride. *Ann Intern Med* 1995; 123:401-8.

27. Wasnich RD, Davis J, Ross P, et al. Effect of thiazide on rates of bone mineral loss: A longitudinal study. *Br Med J* 1990; 301:1303-5.

28. Wasnich RD, Benfante RJ, Yano K, et al. Thiazide effect on the mineral content of bone. *N Engl J Med* 1983; 309:344-7.

29. Ray WA, Griffin MR, Downey W, et al. Long-term use of thiazide diuretics and risk of hip fracture. *Lancet* 1989; 1:687-90.

30. LaCroix AZ, Wienpahl J, White LR, et al. Thiazide diuretic agents and the incidence of hip fracture. *N Engl J Med* 1990; 322:286-90.

31. Felson DT, Sloutskis D, Anderson JJ, et al. Thiazide diuretics and the risk of hip fracture: Results from the Framingham study. *JAMA* 1991; 265:370-3.

32. Heidrich FE, Stergachis A, Gross KM. Diuretic drug use and the risk for hip fracture. *Ann Intern Med* 1991; 115:1-6.

33. Lindsay R, Marshall B, Haboubi A, et al. Increased axial bone mass in women with hypertension: Role of thiazide therapy (abstract). *J Bone Miner Res* 1987; 2 (suppl 1):S29.

34. Morton DJ, Barrett-Connor EL, Edelstein SL. Thiazides and bone mineral density in elderly men and women. *Am J Epidemiol* 1994; 139:1107-15.

35. Whiting SJ. Safety of some calcium supplements questioned. *Nutr Rev* 1994; 52:95-105.

36. Bourgoin BP, Evans DR, Cornett JR, Lingard SM, Quattrone AJ. Lead content in 70 brands of dietary calcium supplements. *Am J Public Health* 1993; 83:1155-60.

Chapter Eight: The Lifestyle Factors: Personal Choices in Everyday Life

1. Cigarette smoking among adults—United States, 1992, and changes in the definition of current cigarette smoking. *Morb Mortal Wkly Report* 1994; 43:342-6.

2. Cigarette smoking among women of reproductive age—United States, 1987–1992. *Morb Mortal Wkly Report* 1994; 43:789-91, 797.

3. US Department of Health and Human Services. *Preventing Tobacco Use among Young People: A Report of the Surgeon General.* Atlanta: USD-HHS, PHS, CDC, 1994.

4. Baron JA, La Vecchia C, Levi F. The antiestrogenic effect of cigarette smoking in women. *Am J Obstet Gynecol* 1990; 162:502-14.

5. Schectman G, Byrd JC, Hoffmann R. Ascorbic acid requirements for smokers: Analysis of a population survey. *Am J Clin Nutr* 1991; 53:1466-70.

6. Midgette AS, Baron JA. Cigarette smoking and the risk of natural menopause. *Epidemiology* 1990; 1:474-80.

7. Jensen J, Christiansen C. Effects of smoking on serum lipoproteins and bone mineral content during postmenopausal hormone replacement therapy. *Am J Obstet Gynecol* 1988; 159:820-5.

8. Byrjalsen I, Haarbo J, Christiansen C. Role of cigarette smoking on the postmenopausal endometrium during sequential estrogen and progestogen therapy. *Obstet Gynecol* 1993; 81:1016-21.

9. Egger P, Duggleby S, Hobbs R, Fall C, Cooper C. Cigarette smoking and bone mineral density in the elderly. *J Epidemiol Community Health* 1996; 50:47-50.

10. Cooper C, Barker DJP, Wickham C. Physical activity, muscle strength, and calcium intake in fracture of the proximal femur in Britain. *B Med J* 1988; 297:1443-6.

11. Hollenbach KA, Barrett-Connor E, Edelstein SL, Holbrook T. Cigarette smoking and bone mineral density in older men and women. *Am J Public Health* 1993; 83:1265-70.

12. Feitelberg S, Epstein S, Ismail F. Deranged bone mineral metabolism in chronic alcoholism. *Metabolism* 1987; 36:322-6.

13. Moniz C. Alcohol and bone. *Br Med Bull* 1994; 50:67-75.

14. Walker ARP. Certain biochemical findings in man in relation to diet. *Ann NY Acad Sci* 1958; 69:989-1008.

15. Modlin M. Urinary calcium in normal adults and in patients with renal stones: An interracial study. *Invest Urol* 1967; 5:49-57.

16. Lynch SR, Berelowitz I, Seftel HC, et al. Osteoporosis in Johannesburg Bantu males. *Am J Clin Nutr* 1967; 20:799-807.

17. Bikle DD, Genant HK, Cann C, Recker RR, Halloran BP, Strewler GJ. Bone disease in alcohol abuse. *Ann Intern Med* 1985; 103:42-8.

18. Frezza M, di Padova C, Pozzato G, et al. High blood alcohol levels in women: The role of decreased gastric alcohol dehydrogenase activity and first-pass metabolism. *N Engl J Med* 1990; 322:95-9.

19. Ashley MJ, Olin JS, le Riche WH, et al. Morbidity in alcoholics: Evidence for accelerated development of physical disease in women. *Arch Intern Med* 1977; 137:883-7.

20. Saunders JB, Davis M, Williams R. Do women develop alcoholic liver disease more readily than men? *Br Med J* 1981; 282:1140-3.

21. Norton R, Batey R, Dwyer T, MacMahon S. Alcohol consumption and the risk of alcohol-related cirrhosis in women. *Br Med J* 1987; 295:80-5.

22. Urbano-Márquez A, Estruch R, Fernández-Solá J, Nicolás JM, Paré JC, Rubin E. The greater risk of alcoholic cardiomyopathy and myopathy in women compared with men. *JAMA* 1995; 274:149-54.

23. Emanuelle N, Emanuelle MA. The endocrine system: Alcohol alters critical hormonal balance. *Alcohol Health Res World* 1997; 21:53-64.

24. Klein RF. Alcohol-induced bone disease: Impact of ethanol on osteoblast proliferation. *Alcoholism Clin Exp Res* 1997; 21:392-9.

25. Sampson HW. Alcohol, osteoporosis, and bone regulating hormones. *Alcoholism Clin Exp Res* 1997; 21:400-3.

26. USDA and USDHHS. *Nutrition and Your Health: Dietary Guidelines for Americans.* 4th edition. Home and Garden Bulletin, 1995.

27. Heaney RP, Recker RR. Effects of nitrogen, phosphorus, and caffeine on calcium balance in women. *J Lab Clin Med* 1982; 99:46-55.

28. Yano K, Heilbrun LK, Wasnich RD, Hankin JH, Vogel JM. The relationship between diet and bone mineral content of multiple skeletal sites in elderly Japanese American men and women living in Hawaii. *Am J Clin Nutr* 1985; 42:877-88.

29. Massey LK, Wise KJ. The effect of dietary caffeine on urinary excretion of calcium, magnesium, sodium, and potassium in healthy young females. *Nutr Res* 1984; 4:43-50.

30. Harris SS, Dawson-Hughes B. Caffeine and bone loss in healthy post-menopausal women. *Am J Clin Nutr* 1994; 60:573-8.

31. Barger-Lux MJ, Heaney RP, Stegman MR. Effects of moderate caffeine intake on the calcium economy of premenopausal women. *Am J Clin Nutr* 1990; 52:722-5.

32. Lloyd T, Rollings N, Eggli DF, Kieselhorst K, Chinchilli VM. Dietary caffeine intake and bone status of postmenopausal women. *Am J Clin Nutr* 1997; 65:1826-30.

33. Packard PT, Recker RR. Caffeine does not affect the rate of gain in spine bone in young women. *Osteoporos Int* 1996; 6:149-52

Chapter Nine: The Nutrient Factors: Translating Research Into Reality

1. US Dept. Agriculture, Economic Research Service. *Food Consumption, Prices, and Expenditures, 1996: Annual Data.* Statistical Bulletin No. 928, April 1, 1996.

2. Murphy SP, Rose D, Hudes M, Viteri FE. Demographic and economic factors associated with dietary quality for adults in the 1987-88 Nationwide Food Consumption Survey. *J Am Diet Assoc* 1992; 92:1352-7.

3. Albertson AM, Tobelmann RC, Engstrom A, Asp EH. Nutrient intakes of 2- to 10-year-old American children: 10-year trends. *J Am Diet Assoc* 1992; 92:1492-6.

4. US Dept. Health and Human Services. *Healthy People 2000. National Health Promotion and Disease Prevention Objectives.* Washington, DC. DHHS Pub No 91-50212, 1990.

5. US Dept. Agriculture, US Dept Health and Human Services. *Nutrition and Your Health: Dietary Guidelines for Americans.* 4th ed. Washington, DC, Home and Garden Bulletin No. 232, 1995.

6. Krebs-Smith SM, Cook A, Subar AF, Cleveland L, Friday J. US adults' fruit and vegetable intakes, 1989 to 1991: A revised baseline for the Healthy People 2000 objective. *Am J Public Health* 1995; 85:1623-9.

7. Albertson AM, Tobelmann RC. Consumption of grain and whole-grain foods by an American population during the years 1990 to 1992. *J Am Diet Assoc* 1995; 95:703-4.

8. Norris J, Harnack L, Carmichael S, Pouane T, Wakimoto P, Block G. US trends in nutrient intake: The 1987 and 1992 National Health Interview Surveys. *Am J Public Health* 1997; 87:740-6.

9. Daily dietary fat and total food-energy intakes: Third National Health and Nutrition Examination Survey, Phase 1, 1988-91. *Morb Mortal Wkly Report* 1994; 43:116, 117, 123-5.

10. Hampl JS, Betts NM. Comparisons of dietary intake and sources of fat in low- and high-fat diets of 18- to 24-year olds. *J Am Diet Assoc* 1995; 95:893-7.

11. Kennedy E, Goldberg J. What are American children eating? Implications for public policy. *Nutr Rev* 1995; 53:111-126.

12. Dehkordi N, Rao DR, Warren AP, Chawan CB. Lactose malabsorption as influenced by chocolate milk, skim milk, sucrose, whole milk, and lactic cultures. *J Am Diet Assoc* 1995; 95:484-6.

13. Solomon NW, Guerro AM, Torun B. Dietary manipulation of postprandial colonic lactose fermentation. I. Effect of solid food in a meal. *Am J Clin Nutr* 1985; 41:199-208.

14. Martin MC, Savaiano DA. Reduced intolerance symptoms from lactose consumed during a meal. *Am J Clin Nutr* 1988; 47:57-60.

15. Martini MC, Kukielka D, Savaiano DA. Lactose digestion from yoghurt: Influence of a meal and additional lactose. *Am J Clin Nutr* 1991; 53:1253-8.

16. Kerstetter JE, Insogna K. Do dairy products improve bone density in adolescent girls? *Nutr Rev* 1995; 53:328-332.

17. Stracke H, Renner E, Knie G, Leidig G, Minne H, Federlin K. Osteoporosis and bone metabolic parameters in dependence upon calcium intake through milk and milk products. *Eur J Clin Nutr* 1993; 47:617-622.

18. Sandler RB, Slemenda CW, LaPorte RE, et al. Postmenopausal bone density and milk consumption in childhood and adolescence. *Am J Clin Nutr* 1985; 42:270-4.

19. Soroko S, Holbrook TL, Edelstein S, Barrett-Connor E. Lifetime milk consumption and bone mineral density in older women. *Am J Public Health* 1994; 84:1319-1322.

20. Matkovic V, Ilich JZ. Calcium requirements for growth: Are current recommendations adequate? *Nutr Rev* 1993; 51:171-180.

21. Matkovic V, Kostial K, Simonovic I, Buzina R, Brodarec A, Nordin BEC. Bone status and fracture rates in two regions of Yugoslavia. *Am J Clin Nutr* 1979; 32:540-9.

22. Halioua L, Anderson JJB. Lifetime calcium intake and physical activity habits: Independent and combined effects on the radial bone of healthy premenopausal Caucasian women. *Am J Clin Nutr* 1989; 49:534-41.

23. Nieves JW, Golden AL, Siris E, Kelsey JL, Lindsay R. Teenage and current calcium intake are related to bone mineral density of the hip and forearm in women aged 30-39 years. *Am J Clin Nutr* 1995; 141:342-51.

24. Massey LK, Whiting SJ. Dietary salt, urinary calcium, and kidney stone risk. *Nutr Rev* 1995; 53:131-9.

25. Whiting SJ. The inhibitory effect of dietary calcium on iron bioavailability: A cause for concern? *Nutr Rev* 1995; 53:77-80.

26. Reddy MB, Cook JD. Effect of calcium intake on nonheme-iron absorption from a complete diet. *Am J Clin Nutr* 1997; 65:1820-5.

27. Wood RJ, Zheng JJ. High dietary calcium intakes reduce zinc absorption and balance in humans. *Am J Clin Nutr* 1997; 65:1803-9.

28. Gleerup A, Rossander-Hulthén, Gramatkovski E, Hallberg L. Iron absorption from the whole diet: Comparison of the effect of two different distributions of daily calcium intake. *Am J Clin Nutr* 1995; 61:97-104.

29. Heaney RP. Lifelong calcium intake and prevention of bone fragility in the aged. *Calcif Tissue Int* 1991; 49: S42-S45.

30. Jackman LA, Millane SS, Martin BR, et al. Calcium retention in relation to calcium intake and postmenarcheal age in adolescent females. *Am J Clin Nutr* 1997; 66:327-33.

31. Matkovic V, Heaney RP. Calcium balance during human growth: Evidence for threshold behavior. *Am J Clin Nutr* 1992; 55:992-6.

32. Baran D, Sorensen A, Grimes J, et al. Dietary modification with dairy products for preventing vertebral bone loss in premenopausal women: A three-year prospective study. *J Clin Endocrinol Metab* 1989; 70:264-70.

33. *Optimal Calcium Intake.* NIH Consensus Statement 1994. June 6-8; 12(4):1-31.

34. National Research Council. *Recommended Dietary Allowances.* 10th edition. Washington, DC: National Academy Press, 1989.

35. Food and Nutrition Board, Institute of Medicine. *Dietary Reference Intakes for Calcium, Phosphorus, Magnesium, Vitamin D, and Fluoride.* Washington, DC: National Academy Press, 1997.

36. Johnston CC, Miller JZ, Slemenda CW, et al. Calcium supplementation and increases in bone mineral density in children. *N Engl J Med* 1992; 327:82-7.

37. Heaney RP. Bone mass, nutrition, and other lifestyle factors. *Nutr Rev* 1996; 54:S3-S10.

38. Chapuy MC, Arlot ME, Duboeuf F, et al. Vitamin D3 and calcium to prevent hip fractures in elderly women. *N Engl J Med* 1992; 327:1637-42.

39. Heaney RP, Recker RR, Stegman MR, Moy AJ. Calcium absorption in women: Relationships to calcium intake, estrogen status, and bone age. *J Bone Miner Res* 1989; 4:469-75.

Chapter Ten: The Food Factors: The Best Choices for Good Health

1. Murphy SP, Rose D, Hudes M, Viteri FE. Demographic and economic factors associated with dietary quality for adults in the 1987-88 Nationwide Food Consumption Survey. *J Am Diet Assoc* 1992; 92:1352-7.

2. Norris J, Harnack L, Carmichael S, Pouane T, Wakimoto P, Block G. US trends in nutrient intake: The 1987 and 1992 National Health Interview Surveys. *Am J Public Health* 1997; 87:740-6.

3. Albertson AM, Tobelmann RC, Engstrom A, Asp EH. Nutrient intakes of 2- to 10-year-old American children: 10-year trends. *J Am Diet Assoc* 1992; 92:1492-6.

4. Mandatory nutrition labeling—FDA's final rule. *Nutr Rev* 1993; 51:101-5.

5. *Federal Register.* January 6, 1993, vol. 58 (3), book II, pp 2665-2681. Rf: HHS FDA 21 CFR.

6. Kreuter MW, Brennan LK, Scharff DP, Lukwago SN. Do nutrition label readers eat healthier diets? Behavioral correlates of adults use of food labels. *Am J Prev Med* 1997; 13(4): 277-83.

Glossary of Terms

active load: the force transmitted to the bones through muscle contraction

alendronate: a drug that slows down bone resorption, also known as Fosamax

anorexia nervosa: an eating disorder characterized by an obsession to be thin and an aversion to food

athletic amenorrhea: the cessation of menstrual periods secondary to intense physical training and reduction in percent body fat

basal metabolic rate: the rate at which we burn calories at rest

binding agents: dietary factors such as oxalates, phytates, phosphates, and fats, that bind calcium to some degree, preventing it from being absorbed

bisphosphonates: a group of drugs that act specifically at the sites of bone turnover, binding to the osteoclasts (the cells that breakdown bone), inactivating them

bone mass or **bone mineral content:** the amount of bone in our bodies

bone mineral density: the amount of calcium in our bones

bulimia: an eating disorder characterized by episodes of food binging followed by self-induced vomiting and purging

calcitonin: the bone-building hormone from the thyroid gland

calcitriol: the most active form of vitamin D

cortical or **compact bone:** the dense outer layer of bone

critical fracture zone: bone mineral density two standard deviations or more below the mean for normal, healthy young adults

designer estrogens: tissue-specific estrogens that have beneficial effects on bone

dietary fiber: a type of carbohydrate found in certain foods that is not absorbed by the body and passes undigested through the gastrointestinal tract

endometriosis: a condition in which tissue from the lining of the uterus (the endometrium) is found outside the uterus or embedded in other tissues of the body

epiphyseal plates: the area of cartilage at the ends of the long bones, where growth occurs

female-athlete triad: the combination of intense physical training, disturbance of normal hormonal levels, and subsequent loss of bone mass

femoral bone: the bone of the upper leg; the femoral joint is the hip joint, a common area for osteoporotic fracture

HRT (hormone replacement therapy): the replacement of declining hormone levels with estrogen and progestins; prevents the rapid bone loss at menopause

hydroxyapatite: the hard, crystalline mineral salts in bone

hypertension: high blood pressure

hysterectomy: the surgical removal of the uterus

impact load: the force transmitted to the bones with weight-bearing exercise

lactose: the double-ringed carbohydrate found exclusively in milk and milk products

menarche: the initiation of the monthly menstrual periods

menopause: one year after the last menstrual period

negative calcium balance: the condition in which more calcium is being excreted or mobilized than is being absorbed, so that calcium is being drawn from the bones

osteoblasts: specialized bone cells that create the bone framework (collagen) and attract calcium and other minerals to strengthen bones by increasing bone density

osteoclasts: specialized bone cells that break down bone (resorption), dissolving bone and releasing calcium and other minerals into the bloodstream

osteoporosis: an age-related bone disorder characterized by an increased susceptibility to fractures

peak bone mass: the maximum amount of bone present before age-related losses begin around menopause

positive calcium balance: the condition in which more calcium is being absorbed during digestion than is being lost in the urine or via the gastrointestinal tract, so that calcium is being added to the skeleton

pure or *elemental calcium:* the amount of a calcium salt, such as calcium carbonate or calcium citrate, that is pure calcium

scoliosis: curvature of the spine

trabecular or *porous bone:* the spongy inner layer of bones

vertebrae: the spine or backbone

Suggested Readings and Resources

National Organizations

- *American Association of Retired Persons (AARP),* 601 E St., NW, Washington, DC 20049; (202) 434-2277; http://www.aarp.org/.
- *American College of Obstetricians and Gynecologists (ACOG),* 409 12th St, SW, Washington, DC 20024-2188, (202)862-2535
- *American Dietetic Association/ National Center for Nutrition and Dietetics,* Consumer Nutrition Hotline (800) 366-1655
- *Lilly Center for Women's Health,* 1-888-WMN-HLTH
- *National Dairy Council,* 6300 North River Rd, Rosemont, IL 60018-4233, (312) 696-1020
- *National Institute on Aging,* Information Center PO Box 8057, Gaithersburg, MD 20898-8057; (800) 222-2225
- *National Osteoporosis Foundation,* 1150 17th St, NW, Suite 500, Washington, DC 20036; (202) 223-2226 and (800) 464-6700; http://www.nof.org/.

- *North American Menopause Society,* c/o University Hospitals of Cleveland, Department of Obstetrics and Gynecology, 11100 Euclid Ave., Suite 7024, Cleveland, OH 44106; (216) 844-8748; http://www.menopause.org/.
- *Older Women's League (OWL),* 666 11th St, NW, Suite 700, Washington, DC 20001; (202) 783-6686
- *Osteoporosis and Related Bone Diseases Resource Center (ORBD-NRC),* (800) 624-2663; TDD (202) 223-0344

Barbara's Favorite Health and Nutrition Magazines

- *American Health for Women,* PO Box 3017, Harlan, IA 51593; (800) 365-5005
- *Cooking Light,* PO Box 1748, Birmingham, AL 35201; (205) 877-6000
- *Eating Well: The Magazine of Food & Health,* PO Box 54263, Boulder, CO 80322-4263; (800) EAT-WELL
- *Living Fit,* PO Box 37209, Boone IA 50037-2209
- *Shape,* PO Box 37207, Boone, IA 50037-2207; (800) 340-8953
- *Walking: The Magazine of Smart Health and Fitness,* PO Box 5011, Harlan, IA 51593-2511; (800) 829-5585

Barbara's Favorite Health and Nutrition Books

- *Body Defining,* by Ellington Darden. Chicago, IL: Contemporary Books, 1996
- *Body Shaping,* by Michael Yessis. Emmaus, PA: Rodale Press, 1994
- *The Eating Well Recipe Rescue Cookbook,* Charlotte, VT: Eating Well Magazine, 1994
- *New York City Ballet Workout,* by Peter Martins. New York: William Morrow and Company, 1997

Index